Health Care in Peru: Resources and Policy

Health Care in Peru: Resources and Policy

edited by
Dieter K. Zschock

Routledge
Taylor & Francis Group
NEW YORK AND LONDON

First published 1988 by Westview Press

Published 2018 by Routledge
605 Third Avenue, New York, NY 10017
2 Park Square, Milton Park, Abingdon, Oxon OX14 4RN

Routledge is an imprint of the Taylor & Francis Group, an informa business

Library of Congress Cataloging-in-Publication Data
Health care in Peru.
(Westview special studies on Latin America and the Caribbean)
Includes index.
1. Medical care—Peru. 2. Public health—Peru. 3. Medical policy—Peru. I. Zschock, Dieter K. II. Series.
RA395.P4P49 1988 362.1'0985 87-14709

ISBN 13: 978-0-367-01407-0 (hbk)

Contents

List of Tables

Acknowledgments

The Health Sector Analysis of Peru (HSA-Peru), upon which this book is based, was a two-year research effort (1985-86) involving 70 Peruvian and international professionals (see Appendix A). The project was funded by the U.S. Agency for International Development, under a Cooperative Agreement with the State University of New York at Stony Brook.

The HSA-Peru owes its successful implementation to the formal endorsements it received from Peruvian Minister of Health Dr. Carlos Bazán Zender in March, 1985, and subsequently from his successor, Dr. David Tejada de Rivero, in August, 1985. The project also received the endorsement of Dr. José A. Barsallo Burga, President of the Peruvian Institute of Social Security. In the design and implementation of the HSA-Peru, the cooperation of the Pan American Health Organization (PAHO)—initially under the direction of its Representative in Peru, Dr. Humberto de Moraes Novaes, and subsequently under his successor, Ing. Carlos E. Cuneo—was instrumental.

The project also benefitted greatly from the formal participation of two Peruvian institutions of higher education: Cayetano Heredia University (UPCH) and the independent Graduate School of Administration and Management (ESAN), both located in Lima, and from the technical assistance services provided by a U.S. consulting firm, International Resources Group, Ltd. (IRG), of Stony Brook, N.Y.

The HSA-Peru was coordinated by a committee of five professionals, including a Peruvian Coordinator appointed by the Minister of Health. Dr. Julio Castañeda Costa served as Coordinator through July 1985, and was succeeded in August, 1985, by Dr. Walter Torres Zevallos, who served through May, 1986. The other committee members were the representative of UPCH, Dr. David Tejada Pardo; the representative of ESAN, Dr. Cesar Peñaranda Castañeda; the representative of IRG, Dr. Luis Carlos Gómez; and the Stony Brook project director (who also edited this book). This committee had the very able administrative assistance of Ms. Maritza Torres, employed by IRG, and Ms. Ethel R. Carrillo, employed by Stony Brook, as well as the full administrative support of the PAHO representative's staff in Lima.

The HSA-Peru benefitted immeasurably from the vision and continuing active involvement of the USAID project manager in Lima, Ms. Norma J.

Parker. Guidance by the USAID health officer, Ms. Joan La Rosa, and other mission staff in Peru was also most helpful throughout the project's duration. Support services provided by the Research Foundation of the State University of New York (represented by Mr. Eugene Schuler), as signatory of the Cooperative Agreement, were essential to the project's implementation. At Stony Brook, project management was facilitated by Dr. Egon Neuberger, Dean of Social Sciences, and Ms. Lynda Perdoma Ayala, assistant to the project director. Mr. Chandra Shrestha served most capably as research assistant.

The accomplishments of the HSA-Peru owe much to the intellectual contributions made by Dr. Petra Reyes, who participated in the design of the analysis, and later by her replacement, Dr. Luis Carlos Gómez, who advised in the design and implementation of original field research during the project's second phase. In editing this book and in drawing conclusions and recommendations from its individual chapters, the participation of my Stony Brook colleague Dr. Gretchen Gwynne has given all of us as collaborators the benefit of a fresh mind.

Finally, production of the manuscript for publication was financially supported by the State University of New York's Office of International Programs, and by International Resources Group, Ltd.

Dieter K. Zschock

PART ONE

The Context of Health Care Policy in Peru

1

Introduction

Dieter K. Zschock

Peru ranks sixth in *per capita* income among eleven Latin American countries that fall into the World Bank's "lower-middle-income" category (World Bank 1986), but are relatively highly urbanized. Urbanization, however, can be a misleading indicator of development: Peru, despite being the most highly urbanized of these eleven countries, suffers the region's second highest infant mortality rate (over 90 deaths per 1000 live births), and its life expectancy is a relatively low 59 years, in contrast to the Latin American average of 64 years (PAHO 1986). Like most countries in the region, Peru has a mixed system of health care, consisting of services provided through a ministry of health, a social security institute, and a diverse private sector. But of all the countries in Latin America, Peru is probably among the least efficient and least equitable in the use of its health sector resources. To make matters worse, the widespread economic recession of the early 1980s, which caused a sharp decline in Peru's economy, led also to a 20 percent reduction (in real terms) in the country's public health sector expenditures between 1981 and 1984.

While health conditions are precarious for all Peruvians, the health status of the country's children ranks among the worst for children anywhere in Latin America. Despite the government's attempt to expand primary health care (PHC) and increase child survival, Peru's infant mortality rate is 50 percent higher than the Latin American average of 63/1000. Infant mortality among the country's poor ranges from 60/1000 in Lima's sprawling shantytowns to 142/1000 in the remote rural areas. The overall death rate remains relatively high at 11/1000, largely because of high infant and child mortality.

Infants in Peru die primarily of perinatal, respiratory, gastro-intestinal, and immuno-preventable diseases. Together, these four causes account for three-fourths of all deaths among children under one year old. An additional five percent of infant deaths can be directly attributed to nutritional deficiency. Child mortality (1-5 years), while it has declined substantially, remains a problem as well; 65 percent of all diarrheal mortality, for example, occurs in children under 3 years of age. And only 25 percent of Peruvian children had been completely vaccinated against immuno-preventable diseases as of the end of 1984.

Health care represents approximately 4.5 percent of the Peruvian gross domestic product (GDP)—an average of close to US $40 worth of medical attention and pharmaceutical products for each of 19 million Peruvians in 1984. Theoretically, this level of resources allocation to the health sector could provide the entire Peruvian population with adequate primary health care—which has been the government's foremost health sector policy priority since 1980 (Bazan 1985)—plus essential hospital services, *if* medical attention were appropriately organized and distributed. But Peru uses three-fourths of its health sector resources to support expensive urban hospitals, and only one-fourth for lower-cost health centers and health posts providing primary health care to its urban and rural poor. As a result, six million Peruvians—almost a third of the population—have no access to modern health services. The HSA-Peru project, a year-long analysis of Peru's health sector in which 70 Peruvian and foreign professionals participated (see Appendix A) and on which this book is based, makes it quite clear that the government's policy of providing primary health care for all Peruvians is likely to remain an elusive objective—unless the country's leadership gives serious consideration to the findings and recommendations presented in the last chapter of this book.

Health Sector Resources and Population Coverage

Peru's physical health sector resources include some 338 hospitals (containing 30,000 beds), 785 health centers, and 1,925 health posts. The country's medical personnel include approximately 13,500 doctors, 11,000 registered nurses, 2,800 pharmacists, and 28,000 paramedical personnel (1984 estimates). The principal institutional health care providers in the public sector are the Ministry of Health (MOH) and the Institute of Social Security (IPSS). Together with the health services operated by the military, the police, and several large parastatal enterprises, public sector health care resources account for 78 percent of the country's hospital beds, 93 percent of its primary health care facilities, close to half of its medical doctors, and a substantial majority of its nursing and paramedical personnel. All told, public health also accounts for two-thirds of total health sector expenditures (Table 1.1).

The MOH reaches only half of the 60 percent of Peru's total population for whose health care it is directly responsible and accounts for only 27 percent of total health spending. In contrast, IPSS, which is responsible for providing medical care for only 18 percent of the population, accounts for 33 percent of total health sector expenditures. Parastatals and the uniformed forces, which maintain their own exclusive health services, account for another 3 percent of coverage and 6 percent of expenditures.

The private health sector is less easily quantified. If all doctors not primarily employed in public health institutions were included, the number in private practice would be over 50 percent of Peru's doctors. The private sector provides only 18 percent of all hospital beds and four percent of primary health care facilities, but accounts for three-fourths of all pharmaceutical sales. A recent household survey on health (ENNSA 1984) reveals that between one-third and two-thirds of all inhabitants of Peru's major urban areas routinely consult private doctors for their outpatient health care needs.

Together, public and private medical services are financially and geographically accessible to approximately 13 million Peruvians. That leaves some six million people—almost all of them poor and a large percentage of them rural—without access to modern health care.

The present configuration of health care institutions in Peru is a product of past political, social, economic and demographic changes—particularly those that occurred from the late 1960s onward. In 1972, the transfer to the MOH of charity hospitals, which had previously been administered by religious orders and inadequately funded through donations and lottery earnings, placed a significant fiscal burden on the Ministry; since then it has been obliged to support these hospitals from general tax revenues. Shortly thereafter, in 1973, separate blue-collar and white-collar social security organizations were integrated into what was to become the IPSS in 1980. Yet even as the government attempted to centralize and strengthen the MOH and IPSS, the economy's shrinking tax base necessitated a reduction in the level of MOH funding.

As inflation, starting in the late 1970s, combined with the economic crisis of 1981-1984, MOH and IPSS spending on health care declined drastically, from US $542 million to US $441 million (as is shown in Table 1.1). With the resulting curtailment of public health services, Peruvians shifted more and more to private medical care. Increased foreign aid disbursements and strengthened technical assistance softened the negative effect of the recession on public health, but well-intentioned efforts to orient the MOH away from hospital-centered services and toward primary health care inevitably failed as medical personnel fought to protect their wages, and deteriorating physical facilities and pharmaceuticals supplies made adequate medical attention increasingly difficult. In the face of shrinking financial resources, hospitals operated by the MOH in the principal urban areas frustrated the joint efforts of the MOH and foreign donors to broaden access to primary health care. As unemployment rose, social security revenues for the IPSS medical care program shrank even more drastically than MOH revenues, and many employers—including the government as employer—failed to pay their mandated contributions to IPSS, a predicament that contributed to increased demand both for the Ministry's urban hospital services and for private sector alternatives.

The use of public and private health services in Peru is overlapping. Especially in the urban areas, households' choices between public and private care depend on income, the perceived severity of illness, the perceived quality of care, and residential proximity to medical care providers. Households generally prefer private practitioners for normal ambulatory treatment—depending, of course, on availability and cost: the higher the level of household income, the more likely it is that private care will be chosen (a preference somewhat stronger for adult than for child care, especially at lower levels of income). Lower-income families in the major urban areas who cannot afford private care tend to seek ambulatory care at public hospitals rather than at primary health care facilities, since for many urban residents PHC facilities are not as readily accessible as hospitals and tend to offer more limited services. Most of the 13 million Peruvians with access to modern health care in either the public or private sector must purchase most of the medicines they consume directly from private pharmacies.

Private health insurance programs emerged in Peru in the mid-1970s, and prepaid plans managed by employers or providers are of even more recent origin. Today, of the estimated four million Peruvians who rely primarily on health services provided by the private sector, 500,000 pay for all their medical services directly, while another three and a half million are covered under various health insurance and prepaid health plans (300,000), by cooperatives (one million), and by private voluntary organizations (PVOs) (2.2 million). Urban cooperatives and PVOs probably cover, for the most part, middle- to lower-middle income segments of the population. These organizations either require prepayment through membership dues (cooperatives) or substantial user fees (PVOs), in return for which their beneficiaries expect the quality of care that they associate with medical doctors and adequate drug supplies. The population served by both types of organizations probably includes a substantial number of households whose heads may be covered by IPSS but whose dependents are not.

Between them, cooperatives and PVOs spend close to US $50 million annually (or about seven percent of total health sector expenditures) on health services, and provide medical services for about 2.2 million urban and one million rural residents—the equivalent of about 17 percent of total health sector coverage (1). Urban cooperatives (mostly savings and loan associations) reimburse their members for both ambulatory and inpatient hospital care. PVOs, in contrast, emphasize primary health care. In most cases they do not provide hospital services, referring patients to public hospitals instead.

In the calculation of the private health sector expenditure total of US $245 shown in Table 1.1, the six million very poor Peruvians who are beyond the current reach of modern medical services and who most probably resort to traditional health care are also included. Their household expenditures for health care are estimated at a total of US $25 million, or $4 *per capita* annually (the equivalent of about 3 percent of the average rural *per capita* income in Peru). In addition, private sector pharmaceutical sales totaling US $145 million must be added. The composition of private sector coverage and expenditures is summarized in Table 1.2. Finally, a composite of all public and private health care coverage and expenditures in Peru is presented in Table 1.3, and the underlying data sources and estimates are explained in Appendix B.

The year during which most of the research for this book was carried out, 1985, was the first full year of economic recovery for Peru. It was also a year of profound political change, as the APRA party, for the first time in its history, gained the presidency, and—in coalition with an alliance of leftist parties—also controlled the Peruvian legislature. Health care became a renewed political priority, and the new government's health sector policy gained quick passage in the legislature with a commitment to increase, by about 50 percent, the proportion of the central government budget allocated to the MOH (*El Peruano* 1985). It was inevitable, however, that this dramatic policy emphasis on public health would confront the reality of firmly entrenched resource allocation patterns.

The Health Sector Analysis of Peru

In 1985, challenged by the premise that the inefficient and inequitable organization and distribution of theoretically adequate health care resources was the main reason why almost a third of the Peruvian population had no access to modern health care, the Peruvian MOH and IPSS invited the State University of New York at Stony Brook, in cooperation with the Pan American Health Organization (PAHO), to organize a study of the country's health sector, the Health Sector Analysis of Peru (HSA-Peru). The study's primary functions would be twofold: to document the disparities between intention and reality within the Peruvian health sector, and to provide an analytical basis for future health sector policy formulation. Rather than focusing primarily on the MOH and its efforts to promote primary health care, the HSA-Peru would provide an overview of the entire health sector, addressing the population's health status; the quantity and distribution of physical facilities, medical personnel and pharmaceuticals; and the financing of the principal providers of health care.

The HSA-Peru was funded by the US Agency for International Development (USAID), which—as the major source of foreign aid for health care development in Peru—shared with the MOH the view that an in-depth analysis of the major factors of production and institutional mechanisms of health care delivery in Peru was needed in order to identify the obstacles impeding the government's long-standing policy commitment to primary health care expansion. Work on the project began in February of 1985.

In July, 1985, when Alan Garcia replaced Fernando Belaunde Terry as President of Peru, he appointed David Tejada de Rivero as Minister of Health. Dr. Tejada, who as Deputy Director of the World Health Organization had helped draft the 1978 Declaration of Alma Ata endorsing "Health for All by the Year 2000" as a universal policy objective, concurred with the premises of the HSA-Peru, and approved the study's continuation. A year later, in July of 1986, he accepted the project's completed series of technical reports as they were originally produced in Spanish and published by PAHO in Lima (ANSSA-Peru 1986a-q); in February 1987, USAID accepted the subsequently-produced series of HSA-Peru technical reports in English (HSA-Peru 1986a-i).

These endorsements of the HSA-Peru owe as much to the process by which the project was conducted as to its findings. Between March 1985 and February 1986, the study's participants assembled a massive information base, analyzed the data it contained, and discussed its policy implications at over a hundred small working group sessions, four two-day workshops, and a final national conference. The findings and recommendations of the HSA-Peru thus reflect the intensive participation of a cross-section of Peruvian experts and their international advisors. This book, however, does not represent a consensus of opinion so much as an informed contribution toward a realistic interpretation of Peruvian health sector problems.

The substantive findings of the HSA-Peru, primarily covering the period 1980-84, remained unchanged for purposes of this book, although the analysis has been reshaped to make the material more cohesive and less technical. Each of the following eight chapters examines an important aspect of health care in Peru in considerable depth, based on intensive analysis of data from Peruvian sources. We believe that the rich database created for the HSA-Peru is entirely sufficient for an analysis of why the apparently adequately endowed Peruvian health sector has failed to serve the entire population.

In Chapter 2, the Peruvian population's health status is profiled by combining data from national census and household survey sources, from hospital and health center records, and from civil registries. Although such epidemiological information is frequently dismissed as being outdated and unreliable, Chapter 2 shows that, by comparing and to some extent combining existing databases and using appropriate interpretive and projective techniques, historical data sets can be brought up to date and adjusted for underreporting, and a reliable rank-ordering of causes of illness and death by age, sex, and geopolitical regions can be prepared. The chapter thus illustrates how incomplete and apparently unreliable health status data, typical of any developing country, can be used as a basis for health planning and decision-making about resources allocation in the health sector.

The formal health sector in Peru is supplemented by informal, community-based, self-help health care efforts. Chapter 3 shows how the deterioration of the country's formal economic and social infrastructure has caused communities to turn to self-help initiatives to meet basic economic and social needs. The government has tended to encourage community participation in health, as have PVOs and cooperatives, but the way such participation is implemented largely determines the success or failure of community-based health projects. A review of past Peruvian experiences with community-based health projects shows that community participation is apt to be ineffective when new administrative structures, in competition with existing political power bases, are imposed from outside. It is much more effective when it originates from within communities and makes use of existing social-organizational structures.

As poor Peruvians in urban slums have resorted to communal self-help in response to the deterioration of formal institutional structures, so the urban middle-class has increasingly resorted to private sector health care alternatives with the deterioration of public health services. Chapter 4 outlines an emerging system of prepaid medical care, including health insurance and other risk-sharing mechanisms, in the Lima/Callao metropolitan area. Medical doctors in private practice are abundantly available, in the capital as well as in other urban areas, on a fee-for-service basis; however, even middle-income Peruvians often cannot afford to pay the required fees, so that most doctors do not earn enough from fees to invest in more than the minimum in equipment and supplies needed to provide ambulatory care. This impasse has given rise to organized medical attention, using group insurance and self insurance mechanisms through employers as well as prepaid plans offered by a few large private clinics and hospitals.

Next, Chapter 5 analyzes the distribution of health care facilities in Peru, and finds that it bears little relation to population distribution. This is true not only for the health sector as a whole, but especially for the MOH. For the first time in Peru, the HSA-Peru related the location of MOH hospitals, health centers, and health posts to population distribution by health region and hospital area (as these existed in 1985). Only then was it possible to calculate ratios of hospital beds and primary health care facilities to population, Using hospital bed occupancy and length-of-stay data, it was also possible to show that Peru's urban areas have significant excess hospitalization capacity due to duplication of facilities among the subsectors, while most smaller towns and rural areas are undersupplied with hospital beds. Considering the distances involved, neither the referral of seriously ill patients from primary care facilities to urban hospitals nor the supervision of primary health care from distant hospital centers—both envisioned under the current organizational system—can possibly work.

Neither is the location of doctors in Peru determined by population distribution or health needs, but rather by the location of the medical schools they attended and the hospitals at which they practice. The analysis of doctor location presented in Chapter 6 is based on records of doctors from the registry of the Peruvian Medical Association (*Colegio Medico*), combined with data from voter registration files and the 1981 national census. For a sample drawn from this combined database, doctors' demographic characteristics (age, sex, and place of birth) were matched with their places of medical education, subsector of primary employment (MOH, IPSS, or other public or private), and current residence. Although the database lacks information on income (a significant determinant of location) and does not account for professional employment in more than one health subsector (information that is currently unattainable), it is nevertheless helpful in identifying several important determinants of doctor location.

In addition to facilities and doctors, pharmaceutical products are a third essential ingredient of modern medical attention. In the absence of data on the distribution of medicines in Peru in relation to population distribution, Chapter 7 instead analyzes the structure of the Peruvian pharmaceuticals market. It shows that three-fourths of all drugs produced in Peru are sold through private pharmacies, and that the public sector's essential medicines program, combined with MOH price controls on private sector sales, has contributed to the sharp decline in Peruvian pharmaceuticals production in recent years. With drugs in short supply in MOH and IPSS facilities, effective medical attention in the public sector depends largely on the ability of patients to buy medicines in the private sector—which further limits the usefulness of public health care to the poor.

Between them, the MOH and IPSS account for 60 percent of all Peru's health sector expenditures (see Table 1.1), as detailed in Chapters 8 and 9, respectively. The Ministry's 27 percent of total health sector expenditures is clearly insufficient to operate 54 percent of the country's hospital beds and 86 percent of its primary health care facilities. The MOH is thus incapable of executing its legal responsibility to provide access to health care for all medically indigent Peruvians. As long as the Ministry remains the country's principal provider of hospital services and is unable to support even its current number of health centers and posts adequately, it cannot expand its primary health services.

On the other hand, IPSS—with only 15 percent of all hospital beds and a mere two percent of primary health care facilities—is comparatively well financed. In contrast to the MOH, which is funded largely from general tax revenues, IPSS (a semi-autonomous dependency of the MOH) operates with revenues from wage-based contributions by employers and employees. It pays higher wages and has better facilities and equipment than the MOH, but because of the failure of employers (including the government) to pay their mandated contributions, in combination with inefficient management, IPSS coverage—primarily employed adults, with only limited services for dependents—is less extensive than it could be.

These eight chapters illustrate, in considerable quantitative detail, that at present the Peruvian health sector is inappropriately structured to fulfill the government's policy of providing "health for all," and is likely to remain so—unless it is substantially reorganized for greater efficiency and greater equality of health care delivery. Chapter 10, after synthesizing the major conclusions of these separate analyses, offers a number of far-reaching recommendations—addressed to the government of Peru, foreign aid donors, and private health sector leaders—that can help bring the allocation of health sector resources into line with the country's health care policy, thus making primary health care and essential hospital services accessible to all Peruvians.

Footnote

1. Information on health care expenditures and coverage by cooperatives and PVOs is based on estimates from two earlier exploratory studies (Burns and Prentice 1983; Keaty and Keaty 1983), although these authors' estimates of health care coverage by cooperatives and of health care expenditures by PVOs have been adjusted downward (see Appendix B).

TABLE 1.1

Composition of Health Sector Expenditures, 1980-84
(totals in millions of U.S. dollars)

Subsector	1980 Total	1980 %	1981 Total	1981 %	1982 Total	1982 %	1983 Total	1983 %	1984 Total	1984 %
Ministry of Health	232.5	32.0	237.7	29.3	212.8	26.9	201.0	28.3	200.7	27.4
Social Security	232.9	32.1	304.2	37.4	301.4	38.0	229.4	32.3	240.5	32.9
Other, public	50.9	7.0	52.9	6.5	51.6	6.5	45.0	6.3	45.7	6.2
Subtotal, public	516.3	71.1	594.8	73.2	565.7	71.4	475.4	66.9	486.9	66.5
Private sector	209.3	28.9	217.6	26.8	226.6	28.6	235.6	33.1	245.0	33.5
Health sector total	725.6	100.0	812.5	100.0	792.4	100.0	711.1	100.0	731.8	100.0

Note: Ministry of Health and Institute of Social Security data were provided by these organizations' budget offices, with totals in soles calculated using Central Bank deflator. Estimates of private sector health care expenditures were taken from Table 1.2. Social Security expenditures for medical care were taken from HSA-Peru 1986h, Table 13, and converted to constant soles. However, the expenditure total for 1984 has been increased to correct for a probable underestimate in this source. Constant soles were converted into U.S. dollars at the average annual exchange rate.

TABLE 1.2

Composition of Estimated Private Health Sector Expenditures and Population Coverage, 1984

(expenditures in U.S. dollars)

Composition of sector	Expenditures (thousands)	Coverage (thousands)	Expenditure per capita
A. Medical services			
Direct household expenditures			
Urban, rich	15,000	500	30
Urban, poor	5,000	1,000	5
Rural, poor	20,000	5,000	4
Health insurance	10,750	215	50
Employer and provider plans	4,250	85	50
Cooperatives			
Urban	18,000	900	20
Rural	5,000	100	15
Private voluntary organizations			
Urban	13,000	1,300	10
Rural	9,000	900	10
Subtotal, urban	66,000	4,000	16-17
Subtotal, rural	34,000	6,000	5-6
Total, medical services	100,000	10,000	10
B. Pharmaceuticals			
Sales to households	100,000	13,000	
Sales to providers	45,000		
Subtotal, pharmaceuticals	145,000	13,000	11
Total, A + B	245,000	—	—

Note: See Appendix B for explanation of assumptions underlying coverage and expenditure estimates.

TABLE 1.3

Composite of Estimated Health Sector Expenditures and Population Coverage, 1984
(totals in millions, except expenditures per capita)

	Expenditures (US$)		Population Coverage		Expenditure per capita (US$)
	Total	Percent	Total	Percent	
Public sector, urban					
Ministry of Health	120	16.4	2.0	10.5	60
Social Security.	241	32.9	3.5	18.4	69
Other	46	6.3	0.5	2.6	92
Subtotal, urban	407	55.6	6.0	31.6	68
Public sector, rural					
Ministry of Health	80	10.9	3.0	15.8	27
Public sector, subtotal	487	66.5	9.0	47.4	54
Private sector, urban					
Households, direct	20	2.7	1.5	7.9	13
Third party pmts. (1)	46	6.3	2.5	13.2	18
Subtotal, urban	66	9.0	4.0	21.1	17
Private sector, rural					
Households, direct	20	2.7	5.0	26.3	4
Third party pmts. (1)	14	1.9	1.0	5.3	14
Subtotal, rural	34	4.6	6.0	31.6	6
Private sector, subtotal	100	13.7	10.0	52.6	10
All urban, subtotal	473	64.6	10.0	52.6	47
All rural, subtotal	114	15.6	9.0	47.4	13
Pharmaceuticals	145	19.8	13.0 (2)	68.4	11
Total health sector	732	100.0	19.0	100.0	39

Note: Average per capita expenditures for the 13 million Peruvians who are assumed to have modern health care in either the public or the private sector is US $54 (i.e., US $732 million, minus US $25 that six million urban and rural poor are assumed to have spent on traditional medicines, divided by 13 million).

(1) Third party payments refers to all employer and provider plans, risk-sharing mechanisms, cooperatives, and private voluntary organizations included in Table 1.2.

(2) Pharmaceuticals sold through the private sector are assumed to be unaffordable for six million Peruvians who are not covered by modern medical services but who are included in total coverage, on the assumption that they are making expenditures for traditional health services.

2

Health Status of the Peruvian Population

Luis Carlos Gómez

Compared to other countries in Latin America, the overall health status of the Peruvian population is poor (Table 2.1; PAHO 1986[II]:193 ff.). Although the rates of both illness and death have declined somewhat in recent years, average infant mortality is still relatively high, between 90 and 100 per 1000 live births (Table 2.2), and in some rural areas reaches as high as 142/1000 (CNP 1984a). Average life expectancy at birth (58.6 years for 1980-85) is lower than in any other country in the region except Bolivia and Haiti (CELADE 1983), and more than half of all children under six years of age are suffering, to one degree or another, from malnutrition (ANSSA-Peru 1986k). Various demographic, socioeconomic and environmental factors—including poverty, ignorance, high fertility, poor nutrition, and unhealthy environmental conditions—have contributed to this distressing situation.

After a brief demographic profile and discussion of the effects of socio-economic factors on the health of Peruvians, this chapter outlines in detail the health status of the Peruvian population, cross-tabulating data from disparate sources and analyzing morbidity and mortality by age groups, by biological causes, and by regions—taking existing socioeconomic and environmental parameters into account in each case. Next it comments on the degree of coincidence between Peruvians' perceptions of their health problems and their actual health status. The chapter then focuses on infant, child, and maternal morbi-mortality, matters of particular concern to Peruvian health sector policy-makers. Finally, the conclusions section summarizes the chapter's most important findings, and comments on their implications.

Sources and Reliability of Data

Information on the health status of Peruvians is limited, and in some cases is based upon estimates or inferences (PAHO 1986[II]:193). Nevertheless, existing data sets can be combined for reasonably reliable and detailed health status analysis.

Reliable data on demographic, socioeconomic and environmental indicators were drawn from the national population censuses of 1941, 1961, 1972, and 1981. National surveys on fertility (ENAF 1977-78), contraception (ENPA 1981), and nutrition and health (ENNSA 1984), all based on probability samplings and thus widely representative of the population as a whole, provided very precise data at the national and regional levels. Since these data were obtained mainly from interviews, however, they may contain inaccuracies or inconsistencies resulting from faulty memory or varying interpretations of the terms used.

The National Vital Statistical System (VSS) provided civil statistics, of which mortality data from death certificates were the most important. These data presented two problems. First, the lack of an efficient data-processing system meant that 1981 data were the latest available, although since significant change in causes of mortality is apt to be slow, the 1981 data are believed to be appropriate for our purposes. And second, there is a considerable under-recording of deaths in Peru, the magnitude of which emerged when Ministry of Health (MOH) mortality figures were compared with estimates provided by the National Statistical Institute (INE). The overall under-recording rate is about 55 percent—even higher for infants and children.

The under-recording of deaths affects mortality indicators differently. It can affect the death rate substantially, so that when precise estimates of death rates by age groups or by causes are required it is necessary to correct for under-registration. However, since the *proportion* of unrecorded deaths varied little during the study period, we believe the unadjusted mortality rates by cause within each age group presented here provide an acceptable picture of trends. The under-recording differential by age has consequences for the magnitude and structure of overall causes of death, since causes of death change dramatically with age. The solution to this problem was an independent analysis by age group using structure and rank order indicators—less affected than rates by under-recording.

The quality of diagnoses of death is sometimes deduced through the proportions of medically certified deaths. Many deaths that are recorded in Peru are not medically certified. However, for groups of causes and even, in many cases, for specific causes of death within age groups, medically certified and uncertified deaths are similar in order and often in percentage structure, primarily because the most common causes of death in Peru—especially of early and accidental deaths—are as easily identified by non-medical as by medically-trained people; moreover, chronic diseases such as tuberculosis or cancer are likely to have been diagnosed medically before death.

An exception to the general observation that medically certified and uncertified deaths are similar in order and structure is the lack of similarity between certified and non-certified deaths from "ill-defined signs and symptoms," a cause that appears as first or second among the leading uncertified causes of death in all age groups, but as a certified cause—ranking seventh through tenth—in only four age groups. Peru has a relatively low percentage of deaths from this cause. However, the high proportion of deaths in the lowest age groups reported to have been caused by pneumonia and septicemia, and the presence of some viral and bacterial causes of death in the highest age groups, are indicators of deficient diagnosis quality. In these particular cases, the appropriate correction would increase the "ill-defined signs and symptoms" group. In general, the most useful way of handling unspecified or ill-founded diagnoses is by grouping causes of death into relatively large categories, which has been done here.

Data on communicable diseases and on hospitalizations for various illnesses were provided by the MOH through OGIE, its General Information and Statistics Office. Although the most recent hospital discharge information dates to 1981, the slow rate of change in the diagnostic structure of hospital discharges for large groups of causes means that 1981 data are generally acceptable for our purposes. This source, which covers 90 percent of MOH hospitals serving nearly 60 percent of the country's population, gives a view of the most important causes of morbidity requiring heavy health expenses. The quality of hospital discharge diagnoses is usually considered very good, since such diagnoses are carried out under the most favorable technical conditions and usually with proper diagnostic support. Our communicable diseases data are derived from outpatient consultation records, mainly from MOH institutions; the majority of Peru's Social Security and private institutions are not included.

Diagnoses from outpatient records were fairly current (1984) and their quality was acceptable for a general appreciation of the relative importance of communicable diseases and their probable long-term trends. Coverage was good, with 82.5 percent of data on communicable disease coming from health professionals and 18.5 percent from paramedics located in rural and marginal urban areas. Both sources yielded similar rank orders of the leading diseases reportable by law.

The analysis thus brings together three major categories of information: population-based data (censuses and surveys), civil statistics, and the records of health care institutions. Prior to the publication of the HSA-Peru technical report on health status (HSA-Peru 1986b), data from these various sources of information had never been collated, much less cross-checked. The three data sets were found to be quite compatible, and were pooled to produce the structure and rank order data presented in this chapter.

Demographic Profile

Population Numbers and Growth

In 1985 there were just under twenty million Peruvians, a figure that is expected, on the basis of fertility and mortality projections, to grow to approximately 28 million by the year 2000 (INE-CELADE 1983). The birth rate decreased from 47.1 live births per 1000 Peruvians in 1950-55 to 35.3 in 1986, and overall fertility from 6.8 to 4.6 live births per woman of childbearing age during the same period (Table 2.2). But the rate of population growth has not yet slowed appreciably, since a decrease in the gross mortality rate (due mainly to a reduction in infant mortality, caused in turn by the birth rate decrease and other socioeconomic factors) from 21.6 deaths per thousand in 1950-55 to 9.7 in 1986 (Table 2.2), has been sharp enough to offset the decline in the birth rate. In the near future, however, the 2.6 percent annual population growth rate calculated at the time of the last national census (1981) should slow as mortality changes in structure by age and the birth rate continues its decline.

For the year 2000, a birth rate of 26.5/1000 and a fertility rate of 3.3 live births per childbearing female are anticipated (INE-CELADE 1983; INE 1984a). The growth rate may drop to 2 percent by the end of the century (Table 2.2). These figures represent a projected 30 percent drop in fertility resulting from more widespread knowledge and increased use of birth control methods (ENPA 1981). Life expectancy increased from 43.9 years in 1950-55 to 58.6 in 1980-85, and, as of 1984, was expected to reach 60.8 in 1986 (Table 2.2)—a clear indicator of overall health status improvement. It is projected, also based on the hypothetical 33 percent decrease in mortality, that by 1995-2000 the life expectancy at birth of the average Peruvian will be 67 years.

Age/Sex Distribution and Dependency Index

A breakdown of the Peruvian population by age since 1940 reveals a young population, tending to become even younger up to 1972. During the 1940-72 period, the percentage of the population under 15 rose slightly, from 42.1 percent to 43.8 percent, due mainly to high and stable fertility and a decrease in infant mortality (CNP 1984b; INE 1984a). Decreasing fertility since 1972 (Table 2.2), however, has resulted in a reduction in the number of youths under 15 to 41.5 percent of the population in 1981, and it was estimated that in 1986 the figure would be further reduced to 40.2 percent (Table 2.3). In 1981 the dependency index—the ratio of children and elders to working-age people—was 83.2 (quite high for the region), meaning that there were 83 Peruvians either under 15 or over 65 for every 100 in their productive years (Table 2.3).

By the year 2000, a moderate drop in fertility is expected to reduce the percentage of children under 15 to 35.6 percent of the population. In turn, the potential labor force—Peruvians aged 15-65—will increase from 56.2 percent of the population in 1986 to 60.1 percent by the year 2000, and the number of people over 65 will increase from 3.6 to 4.3 percent during the same period (Table 2.3; CELADE 1983). Thus, from 1986 to 2000, the absolute number of Peruvian children under 15 will increase from 8.1 to 9.9 million, despite the decrease in fertility, and the absolute number of adults 65 and over will increase from 728,000 to 1.2 million because of increased life expectancy. In absolute terms, therefore, there will be more dependent Peruvians than ever before—even though the dependency index will have declined to 66.4 per 100 by the year 2000 as the percentage of children declines with the reduced fertility rate.

The ratio of males to females in Peru has remained the same over the last 40 years: approximately 101/100. But male mortality is higher at all ages, and the preponderance of males is eliminated by age 40. From that age onward the number of females exceeds the number of males. This in turn influences the causes of morbi-mortality over that age due to the higher proportion of female problems in women over 40. By age 70, the number of males is reduced to 78 per 100 females (INE 1984a). No changes in the sex structure of the Peruvian population are anticipated for the immediate future.

Urban/Rural and Regional Composition of Population

As in most Latin American countries, there has been significant migration in Peru from rural to urban areas and from smaller to larger communities—particularly to coastal towns and cities. While the overall population grew at an average annual rate of 2.3 percent between 1940-81, the urban growth rate was 3.8 percent and the rural rate only 0.8 percent (Table 2.4). During the same period, the urban proportion of the population climbed from 35.4 percent to 64.8 percent, and will reach an estimated 74.6 percent (27.9 million people) by 2000 (Table 2.4). Major population concentrations are found in Lima/Callao, Arequipa, Ica, and Cuzco.

Despite the recent (though slight) slowdown in the rate of population growth, the process of urbanization in general and the growth of Lima in particular continue to be important features of the Peruvian demographic situation. Migrants, although in fewer numbers, continue to move to Lima and Callao—now home to 29 percent of Peru's population and over half its urban dwellers. Between 1940 and 1961, while the country was growing at an annual rate of 2.2 percent, Lima's population gained 5.1 percent annually, due both to natural growth and rural-urban migration; its growth rate between 1961-1972 rose to 5.5 percent, compared to a 2.9 percent rate of growth for the country as a whole. From 1972 to 1981, however, the rate of increase diminished to 3.7 percent per year (Aramburu 1983:88). Apparently, the city had experienced such a sharp deterioration in living conditions, urban services, and economic opportunities that not only was there a decrease in natural growth, but fewer and fewer people were making the decision to immigrate. The declining expansion of Lima (a pattern repeated in other major Peruvian cities as well) is a clear indication not of an improvement of living conditions in rural areas—indeed, these are substantially worse off than most cities—but of the complete saturation of urban resources.

The three major geographic regions of Peru—the coast, *sierra* and jungle—house unequal proportions of the population. Immigration to the coast, along which Peru's major cities lie, has been heavy in the last 40-50 years. In 1940, for example, this area held only 28.3 percent of the total population; it now houses 50 percent (Table 2.5). The population of the mountainous *sierra* region, on the other hand, has gradually become smaller, down from 65 percent of the total at the time of the 1940 census to only 39.4 percent in 1981. Because of its geography and environment, Peru's jungle region has the lowest proportion of the population—10.6 percent (Table 2.5). However, the last two censuses suggest an upward trend. In 1981, half of the jungle departments showed a positive net migration rate, and the rates for Madre de Dios (23 percent) and Ucayali (13.3 percent) were among the highest in the country (HSA-Peru 1986b:6).

Effects of Social and Environmental Factors on Health Status

There are strong correlations between health status, as reflected by infant and general mortality and life expectancy, and demographic, economic, social, and environmental factors. In Peru, politically divided into 25 departments with pronounced environmental, demographic, economic, and social differences, the departments with the lowest infant and general mortality rates and the highest life expectancies are those with the lowest birth, fertility and illiteracy rates, the highest percentages of surviving children, a smaller number of workers in the primary sector and therefore a higher proportion in the modern sector, a higher GDP, higher proportions of homes with connected utilities, more medical consultations per person, and more favorable ratios of population to hospital beds and physicians (Table 2.6). These departments (including the heavily urban departments of Lima, Callao, Ica, and Arequipa) are concentrated on the coast; departments located entirely in the *sierra*, such as Huancavelica, Cuzco, Ayacucho, Puno, and Apurimac, suffer much worse living conditions—reflected in their high rates of out-migration and low rates of population growth. Living conditions in the jungle departments, such as Amazonas and Ucayali, fall between those of the coast and the *sierra* (Table 2.6).

Since the turn of the century, there have been pronounced imbalances in resources and political power among the various regions and departments in Peru, and today both are concentrated more heavily in the capital than ever before. Lima accounts for 54 percent of GDP, 70 percent of the industrial plants, 99 percent of all private investment, 65 percent of government expenditures, and 82 percent of bank loans (Izquierda Unida 1985:98). This near-monopoly of resources has contributed to the economic decline of rural areas, which have also suffered, since the 1950s, from a general dissolution of the traditional social and economic structures that once provided at least minimal stability. Mortality figures, much lower in urban areas, reflect this increasing rural impoverishment. Life expectancy in Lima (1983) is over 71 years, as compared to 47 for Huancavelica and Cuzco (Table 2.6). General mortality follows the same pattern: Lima's mortality rate is 5.6/1000, in contrast to 19/1000 and 20/1000 (not adjusted by age structure) for Cuzco and Huancavelica respectively. Infant mortality figures reflect an even greater disparity: Lima's rate is 56/1000, while some *sierra* departments, mostly rural, suffer astonishing rates of as high as 142/1000 (Table 2.6).

Morbidity and Mortality

Overview

Based on the data sources described above and detailed in the following sections (sources that discount malnutrition as a cause of illness), Peru's most serious health problems are respiratory ailments and intestinal infections—the first and second leading causes of mortality across all age groups (Table 2.7). Acute respiratory diseases account for half of all ambulatory morbidity in Peruvians over the age of one, and nearly a third of all infant, child, and adolescent deaths (see Tables 2.8 and 2.9). Intestinal infections are the second highest cause of morbi-mortality across all age groups. Together these two categories of disease account for more than 70 percent of all cases of communicable illness in Peru. In children, the proportion is even higher: these ailments, for example, account for 92 percent of illness in children under one.

Other health problems of especially grave concern are infant deaths from perinatal problems, obstetrical problems in women from 15-44, and injuries due to accidents or violence. For infants under the age of one, problems initiated in the perinatal period, which are the leading cause of death, cost more than 8000 infants their lives in 1981, followed by respiratory (over 5000) and intestinal infections (over 3000) (OGIE 1975-81). Although the perinatal deaths category applies only to infants under the age of one, such deaths occur so frequently in Peru that they are the third leading overall cause of death, after respiratory and intestinal infections (Table 2.7). In females between 15-44, obstetrical problems (which do not include normal deliveries) and abortions rank as the first and second leading causes of morbidity based on hospital discharge data. Indeed, obstetrical problems—many of them resulting from medically unsupervised abortion attempts—are so common in Peru that even though they occur only in females of reproductive age they rank as the overall primary cause of hospital discharges (Table 2.7). Accidents and violence also take a heavy toll, killing more Peruvians between the ages of 15-44 than any other cause of death, and ranking third in hospitalizations in the overall population.

Self-perceived Morbidity

In 1984, a probabilistic sample of Peru's population (approximately 100,000 persons in 20,000 households) was surveyed under the Peruvian National Health and Nutrition Survey (ENNSA 1984). Adult respondents were asked to report any illness they believed they had suffered during the two-week period preceding the survey, any inactivity resulting from such illness, and any health services sought and/or received. Mothers were asked to report on illness perceived in their children.

Some symptoms of illness had been perceived by 35.3 percent of the interviewees within the two-week period prior to their interviews (Table 2.10). The most significant symptoms were respiratory problems (16.8 percent of the total number of cases), digestive problems (7.0 percent), dental problems (3.3 percent), and accidents (1.7 percent). The perception of illness varied with age: it was highest among the young (63.4 percent of children under one and 58.8 percent of those 1-4 were perceived to have been ill) and in those over 65 (51.8 percent), and lowest in the 15-24 year age group (18.6 percent). Very young children suffered more perceived illness than any other age group; overall rates of intestinal and respiratory problems were high, with infants under one suffering the highest prevalence of both problems. Women perceived symptoms more frequently (37.7 percent) than did men (33.2 percent). The perception of illness also varied with family income and the educational level of heads of households; it was higher among very low-income respondents (40 percent) and those with little education (35.9 percent), and lower among those with more economic resources (29.5 percent) and education (32.2 percent) (Table 2.8). There was no significant difference in the perception of illness between urban and rural respondents, or between those in one geographical region and another—with one notable exception: while most regions had illness-perception levels of 33 percent and over, the prevalence of perceived illness along the southern coast and in the mountains was only 26 percent, for no immediately apparent reason (although because of random variation the statistical significance of the difference was not tested).

Almost a fifth of the Peruvians who felt they had suffered an illness over the preceding two-week period had been unable to carry out their normal activities because of it. The prevalence of incapacity in adult Peruvians increased with age, from 4.8 percent in the 15-24 age group to 12.9 percent in respondents 65 and over. It declined in relation to family income and the education level of the head of household, and, like perceived illness, was at its lowest level in the southern coastal area (3.9 percent) and the mountain region (4.4 percent). These trends were repeated in all educational and income groups, with much lower incapacity levels in respondents enjoying better cultural and economic conditions.

Together these survey data suggest that Peru should focus attention on the health of children, the elderly, females of childbearing age, and low-income and poorly educated Peruvians over the age of 25.

Communicable Diseases

The Peruvian Ministry of Health's compulsory reporting of 51 communicable diseases covered districts containing 75.4 percent of the Peruvian population in 1984 (OGIE 1970-84). In that year, the incidence of these diseases was 3.9 cases per 100 population, for a total of 753,000 cases. Approximately half of these cases (48.4 percent) occurred in children under five years of age, and two-thirds in those under 15. It should be pointed out that 18.5 percent of these cases were reported not by health professionals but by paramedics, the primary health care personnel in rural and urban marginal areas, although the rank order of diseases reported by these auxiliary health workers was similar to what was reported by health professionals.

The common cold and other acute respiratory diseases caused almost half (46.1 percent) of the cases of illness reported in Peru in that year. When compared to data from previous years, this figure suggests a steady increase in the incidence of these ailments; there were, for instance, 1,334 cases per 100,000 in 1982 and 1,808 per 100,000 in 1984, a 36 percent increase, although part of this increment is attributable to improved records coverage, which was broadened by 4.5 percent during the same period. Gastroenteritis, enteritis, and dysentery ranked second in prevalence, accounting for 24.3 percent of Peruvian communicable diseases. Again, the incidence of these diseases appears to have increased during the 1970-1984 period—at a rate three times higher than the increase in records coverage. However, both the high lineal correlation between incidence and coverage (0.87) and the decline in mortality from these problems suggest that the observed increase in morbidity is due to improvements in the reporting system. Together, respiratory and gastroenteric diseases accounted for nearly three-fourths of all communicable diseases reported for Peru in 1984. Other important diseases—but with much lower incidence—were the parasitic infection helminthiasis (6.5 percent of 1984 cases), malaria (4.5 percent), respiratory tuberculosis (3.0 percent), and typhoid and paratyphoid fever (2 percent) (Table 2.8).

Hospitalizations and Discharges

Bearing in mind the sources and reliability of the data mentioned earlier, hospitalization data (excluding hospitalizations for normal childbirth) provide a complementary indicator of health status, reflecting a population's perceptions of illnesses severe or complex enough to require specialized, expensive treatment. Table 2.11 presents data on hospital discharges from MOH facilities and on the duration of hospitalizations in 1980, allowing one to assess the economic impact of particular causes of morbidity. In 1981, approximately 371,000 Peruvians were hospitalized for illness in MOH hospitals (1) and later discharged. This represents a rate of 2.1 discharges for morbidity causes per 100 people—an increase over the 1977 figure of 1.7 per 100 (MOH 1977-81). The morbidity discharge proportion for children under five, however, declined from 16.8 percent in 1977 to 14.5 percent in 1981. It is pertinent to note here that according to figures supplied by the MOH and the Peruvian Social Security Institute there was a decrease in the ratio of hospital beds to people (HSA-Peru 1986e; see also Chapter 5).

Direct obstetrical problems, on the increase since 1977, represented 16.2 percent of hospital discharges, and were the main cause of hospitalization for morbidity in Peru in 1981 (Table 2.12). (Hospital discharges for normal childbirth were excluded for this part of the analysis.) The length of stay for obstetrical problems was relatively short (7.9 days in 1980), although due to the volume of cases this cause ranked fifth in the total number of person/days of hospitalization in 1980 (Table 2.11). Digestive tract disorders (other than those of the oral cavity), second in number of hospital discharges, also increased, and the average hospital stay for digestive tract problems was twice as long, for a total of 562,000 person/days of hospitalization in 1980. Respiratory infections—the most common communicable diseases in Peru—were a much less significant cause of hospitalization and lost productive time, ranking 6th (Table 2.12). These figures add weight to both the ENNSA self-perception data (Table 2.10) and the pooled morbi-mortality data (Table 2.7), reinforcing the conclusion that obstetrical and digestive problems deserve increased public health attention in Peru.

Hospital discharges by department are shown in Table 2.13. Direct obstetrical problems were first in almost half of the departments, including those with the highest socioeconomic conditions. Abortion placed third to seventh. Accidents and violence placed first in half of the departments, including the most underdeveloped. Digestive tract diseases placed second to fifth, and intestinal infections second to seventh.

Mortality

Recent Peruvian mortality figures since 1975 from the Peruvian Vital Statistical System reflect a level of under-registration varying between a high of 63.9 percent in 1976 and a low of 46.3 percent in 1980 (OGIE 1975-81; INE 1985a). In 1981 (the most recent year for which figures are available), 88,441 deaths were officially recorded in Peru—a figure representing less than half of the estimated number of actual deaths (OGIE 1975-81). Official mortality figures thus yield an inaccurate overall mortality rate of 5.0 deaths per 1000 population; the estimated true rate for 1981 was 12 per 1000. Moreover, the proportion of medically-certified deaths has declined slightly since 1976. Only 62.1 percent of those deaths that were recorded in 1981 were medically certified, as opposed to 67.3 percent in 1976. Nevertheless, it is clear that Peru's overall estimated mortality rate has dropped steadily during the second half of this century, from 21.6 per 1000 in 1950-55 to 11/1000 for 1980-85 (Table 2.2). In addition, the age structure of (registered) deaths has been changing steadily; the proportion of deaths of children under five decreased from 46.3 percent in 1975 to 39.3 percent in 1981, and the proportion of deaths of those 65 years and over increased, in turn, from 23.8 percent in 1975 to 28.6 percent in 1981 (OGIE 1975-81). It is evident that more and more Peruvians are surviving into adulthood.

Peruvian overall mortality data by cause should be interpreted carefully because of the under-registration differential by age and the variety of causes of mortality at different ages. The five leading causes of death registered in 1981 were diseases of the respiratory system, not including common upper-respiratory infections (20.6 percent); intestinal infections (9.1 percent); perinatal problems (8.6 percent); ill-defined signs and symptoms (8.4 percent); and neoplasms (7.7 percent) (Table 2.9). Adjustments for under-registration would significantly increase the proportion of deaths caused by respiratory ailments, intestinal infections, and perinatal problems.

Mortality data by departments clearly reinforce the association of health status with living standards and environmental conditions (see Table 2.14). Respiratory problems were the first-ranking cause of death in 20 of Peru's 25 departments; the exceptions were Callao and Lima, with the best (average) living conditions, and Amazonas, Madre de Dios and Ucayali, located in the jungle region (OGIE 1975-81), whose mortality rates from intestinal and ill-defined problems exceed those from respiratory infections. Intestinal infections appeared among the ten most prevalent causes of death in all departments, with the more underdeveloped departments suffering the highest rates.

Infant, Child, and Maternal Morbi-mortality

Biological Causes of Infant and Child Morbidity and Mortality

Of communicable diseases reported to the MOH by professionals or paramedics in 1984, acute respiratory infections (common colds and others) were the most common cause of illness in Peruvian children under five, accounting for 51.4 percent of communicable diseases reported by professionals in infants under one and 47.4 percent in children 1-4, and 46.6 percent and 39.2 percent of illnesses reported by paramedics for the same age groups (OGIE 1970-84). The total number of reported cases of these diseases in children under five in that year was 171,964, or 45.5 percent of all diseases reported for this population. The gastroenteric diseases—gastroenteritis, enteritis and dysentery—were the second most important group of communicable diseases in children under five. In 1984, 72.1 percent of all cases of gastroenteric disease recorded by professionals and paramedics were in this age group. Together these two categories of disease were responsible for 83.5 percent of all recorded communicable diseases in children under five in 1984 (Table 2.8), and for 40-50 percent of hospital discharges and mortality. Perinatal problems (in children under one) and accidents were the third ranked causes of mortality and hospital morbidity, respectively, in the overall population (Tables 2.9 and 2.12).

Of vaccine-preventable diseases, five of the most prevalent nationwide, as reported by professionals (OGIE 1970-84), were—in rank order—measles, whooping cough, tetanus, diphtheria and acute poliomyelitis (Table 2.15). Measles, the most prevalent vaccination-preventable disease, occurred at rates of 334/100,000 in infants under one year and 260.2/100,000 in children 1-4 in 1984, although these rates fluctuated widely between 1980-84. Whooping cough, the second most prevalent vaccine-preventable illness, decreased between 1980-84 despite increased recording coverage (61.8 percent in 1980 to 75.4 percent in 1984), with a rate of 172/100,000 in infants under one in 1984 and 93.8/100,000 in children 1-4. Tetanus also declined between 1980-84 in infants under one, from 44.6/100,000 in 1980 to 26/100,000 in 1984, despite improved coverage. In children 1-4, however, the number of cases of tetanus varied from year to year; there were almost twice as many cases in 1984 (a rate of 1.3/100,000) as in 1983. The number of cases of diphtheria and polio varied widely. Vaccination coverage, estimated to be medium to low in the 1984 National Health and Nutrition Survey, explains the high rates of measles, whooping cough and tetanus, particularly in infants under one. Despite the fact that they are preventable, then, these diseases still pose a significant health problem in Peru.

Infant Mortality

Peru's estimated infant mortality rate was 98.6 per 1000 live births in 1980-1985. Specific mortality by sex, while somewhat underestimated, is greater among males (95.4/1000) than females (85.3/1000) (INE-CELADE 1983; INE 1984c). This represents an important improvement over the 1950-1955 period, when infant mortality stood at a high 158.6/1000 live births (INE-CELADE 1983). The proportion of infant mortality occurring in the neonatal period (the first month of life) also declined; between 1971-75 it stood at 45.1 percent, but by 1978-84 had dropped to 39.1 percent. Greater rates of infant mortality occur in children of mothers under twenty (110.7/1000) and over 30 (110.2/1000), and there is a marked tendency towards an increase in neonatal mortality in babies born to mothers between 25-29 years (39.2 in 1961-65 and 47.4 in 1971-75) (Ramos 1981).

Neonatal-period and early-infancy illness, relatively equal in Peru, are caused to a great extent by problems initiated in the perinatal period (90 percent), congenital anomalies (4.2 percent) and intestinal infections (3.2 percent). In turn, the most important specific perinatal causes of mortality are hypoxia, asphyxia, and other respiratory diseases of the fetus and newborn (52.6 percent), and slow fetal growth, malnutrition, and fetal immaturity (OGIE 1975-81). A comparison of the *proportion* of infant mortality that occurs in the neonatal period in the Americas places Peru in an intermediate position (OPS 1979; Ramos 1981), although Peru's mortality *rates* for both the neonatal and infancy periods are high.

Socioeconomic correlates of infant mortality include the mother's educational level and the parents' latest jobs (especially the mother's). Indeed, the mother's education is the most important predictive factor in infant mortality (Ramos 1981), although there is also a high correlation between infant mortality and both fertility and employment. Neonatal, postneonatal and infant mortality in 1971-75 were 3.3 times greater in mothers with no education than in those who had attended high school or university (Ramos 1981). Professional and clerical mothers had an infant mortality rate of only 17.4/1000 in 1971-75, while other occupational groups suffered rates of over 100/1000. Cross-tabulating the mother's educational level by region yielded important differences between mothers with no schooling and those with high school educations or more; for example, neonatal mortality on the coast was 4.7 times higher for mothers with no schooling (Ramos 1981).

Regionally, the coast (excluding Lima) had the lowest levels of infant mortality (95.0/1000—neonatal 47.5 and postneonatal 47.5). A cross-tabulation of mortality by region and urbanization revealed some important facts: the urban/rural differential was extremely marked on the coast, medium in the mountains, and minimal in the jungle, with the big coastal towns having the lowest mortality levels and the rural *sierra* the highest. The percentage of infant mortality during the neonatal period tended to decrease with the level of urbanization in all regions (Ramos 1981); estimates based on ENNSA (1984) data establish a rate of 59 deaths per 1,000 live births in metropolitan Lima for the period 1978-84, 88/1000 for other urban areas, and 117/1000 in rural areas (2).

A clear association can be seen between infant mortality and prenatal care, place of birth, type of attention received, and child care provided (3). Considerably lower mortality (40 to 50 percent less) occurred in children of mothers receiving prenatal care and delivery in a health establishment with medical care. Similarly, mortality was lower in infants who received health care during the first months of life and in those who had been vaccinated.

Malnutrition in Children

Although malnutrition does not appear as a cause of illness or death in either health care institutional records or the records of the Peruvian vital statistical system, it is nevertheless an important factor underlying morbi-mortality in Peru, particularly among children. Data on malnutrition in children are available from several important sources: the anthropometric measurements of the 1984 National Health and Nutrition Survey (INE-MOH 1985), in which the specific age groups and regions with the greatest nutritional deficiencies in children under six were identified; the National Survey on Food Consumption (ENCA 1972), which (despite somewhat different analytic parameters) provided baseline data against which changes reflected in the 1984 survey could be measured; and the ANSSA exploratory report on the nutritional status of children under six (ANSSA-Peru 1986k).

Malnutrition in children decreased between the time of the 1972 National Survey on Food Consumption and the 1984 ENNSA survey, with the greatest absolute reductions taking place along the (urban) southern coast, in the northern, central and southern mountain areas, and in the lowland jungle (ANNSA-Peru 1986k). Today, the greatest nutritional deficiencies in children under six are found in rural areas of all regions, with the most severe cases turning up in all mountain regions, where both chronic and overall malnutrition are high. Metropolitan Lima and the south coast have the lowest levels of these types of malnutrition (INE-MOH 1985).

In rural areas of Peru today, serious nutritional deficiencies are reflected in height-by-age data (a sign of chronic malnutrition) and in weight-by-age data (a sign of overall malnutrition, including both chronic and acute problems) in children under six. Malnutrition is a significant cause of morbidity and mortality in Peruvian infants under one (OGIE 1975-81), often manifesting itself in nutritional dwarfism by the sixth month of life, particularly in the northern and central mountain areas (ANNSA-Peru 1986k).

Maternal Morbi-mortality

Special mention should be made of maternal morbidity and mortality resulting from complications related to pregnancy, abortion, childbirth, and the puerperal period. In 1981, these causes produced 573 maternal deaths and almost 100,000 hospital discharges. Although the largest category of maternal hospital discharges in the MOH figures (OGIE 1975-81) was unspecified obstetrical causes, it is clear that significant problems include abortion, which accounted for 34.6 percent of all obstetrical hospital discharges in 1981; obstructed delivery (16.4 percent), hemorrhage during pregnancy or delivery (6.3 percent), and toxemia (3.3 percent). The abortion figure probably reflects significant under-recording.

These figures suggest that maternal health is still a critical problem in Peru. In 1981, a total of 60,091 instances of hospitalization for direct obstetrical causes (excluding normal delivery) and 31,860 for abortions was reported to the

Ministry of Health. These amounted to 42.6 percent of all hospital discharges reported in that year for all causes.

Conclusions

Summary

Acute respiratory diseases are clearly the most important cause of morbidity and mortality in Peru (see Table 2.7). They appear in first place, across all age groups, among self-perceived illnesses as recorded by the National Health and Nutrition Survey, again in first place among the communicable diseases reported by the outpatient departments of MOH health care facilities, and once again in first place among the causes of mortality recorded by Peru's Vital Statistical System. Respiratory infections are among the five leading causes of morbi-mortality in every age group.

For Peruvians of all ages, intestinal infections are the second leading cause of self-perceived morbidity, of communicable disease, and of mortality, and the fifth leading cause of hospitalization. This problem is one of the three most important causes of morbidity and mortality in Peruvians under the age of 15, and the second most frequent communicable disease and self-perceived illness in all age groups over 15 years.

Across the entire population, other ailments, while perhaps not as widespread as respiratory and intestinal problems, still exact a high toll in human suffering. Accidents and violence are important causes of morbidity and mortality in Peruvians of all ages up to 64 years. They are the primary cause of death in those between 15 and 44 years, and the primary cause of hospitalization in the 5-14 age group. Digestive tract diseases other than intestinal problems appear among the five leading causes of hospital discharges in all age groups over one year, and are first in those 45 and over. Malignant neoplasms and heart disease are among the first five causes of morbi-mortality over 45 years, and malaria and tuberculosis appear consistently in all age groups over five years.

A comprehensive look at the causes of morbidity and mortality in Peruvian children under the age of one shows that problems initiated during the perinatal period are the main cause of hospitalization and death for these children. Acute respiratory diseases are the cause of morbidity most often reported both by mothers and by doctors in out-patient services of MOH institutions, and the second most frequent cause of mortality. Intestinal infections rank second as causes of all reported morbidity in this age group. Together, perinatal problems, respiratory diseases, and intestinal infections produced, in 1981, 69.5 percent of hospital discharges and 77.6 percent of deaths in Peruvian children under one.

For children between the ages of 1 and 4, the same problem most commonly afflicting infants—acute respiratory disease—is the leading cause of all reported morbidity and mortality. Intestinal infections rank second in reported morbidity for this age group (as they do for children under one) and second in mortality as well. Viral and bacterial diseases are among the first five causes of death. In the first group, measles and chicken pox account for almost three-quarters of all cases; in the second, whooping cough is particularly important as a cause of morbi-mortality in children under five. Although malnutrition does not appear in institutional records and the vital statistical system, it has a relevant place among the causes of morbi-mortality; ENNSA results demonstrate the very high prevalence of this problem in children under five.

In Peruvian women, problems related to pregnancy, labor and delivery—not counting normal deliveries—account for 44 percent of hospital discharges for the 15-24 age group. Direct obstetrical problems and abortion rank first and second as causes of hospitalization in Peruvians between 15 and 44 years of age. An unknown number of the hospitalizations for direct obstetrical causes are associated with self-induced abortions.

Peruvians' perceptions of their health problems provide an accurate mirror of reality for the most serious problems: respiratory and digestive tract ailments were perceived as the most commonly suffered illnesses. Very young children were perceived to suffer more illness than any other age group, again an accurate reflection of the actual health status of the Peruvian population. The poor and uneducated believe their rates of illness to be somewhat greater than what higher-income, better- educated Peruvians perceive.

Regionally, health status in Peru closely parallels other developmental indicators. The most urban departments, located on the coast, enjoy less infant mortality; longer average life expectancies; lower birth, fertility and mortality rates; and more favorable doctor/patient and hospital/patient ratios than rural departments, especially in the *sierra*.

Implications of Findings

Based on the data presented in this chapter and aggregated in Table 2.7, a number of broad observations can be made about the overall health status of Peruvians and measures that might be taken to improve it.

1. Most of the premature deaths in Peru are the result of preventable causes, whether diseases or accidents; non-preventable ailments, such as congenital abnormalities, heart conditions (partially), or neoplasms, are responsible for relatively little sickness and death among Peruvians under the age of 65. The

extent of illness that might be avoided medically or environmentally suggests an urgent need for expanded health care and social services. In particular, infant mortality, which is strongly correlated with malnutrition, maternal education, and maternal employment status, should be a primary target for improved services.

2. The very high rates of illness and death in Peru from respiratory and intestinal infections—both communicable diseases—and from malnutrition attest to the wide prevalence of sub-standard living and working conditions. The lack of pure water, electrical power, and sewerage, as well as general poverty and maternal educational deficiencies, are strongly correlated with the incidence of these problems.

3. The high proportion of hospitalizations for obstetrical problems among Peruvian women of reproductive age suggest that the rate of ambulatory morbidity due to obstetrical causes must be truly prodigious. This in turn suggests either a severe lack of gynecological education and primary gynecological care or a failure to make use of it. Although the number of obstetrical cases resulting from attempted self-induced abortion is unknown, it is thought to be very high. More gynecological education, particularly in birth control methods, and better access to modern obstetrical care are needed.

4. The high rate of perinatal deaths in Peru reflects environmental (including nutritional) and maternal educational deficiencies, a lack of access to or insufficient health services, or services of a minimum level of quality. Together these problems lead to the inescapable conclusion that maternal and infant health should be matters of urgent priority in Peru.

5. The high number of deaths from "ill-defined symptoms" suggests that diagnoses may be of poor quality, that there is a widespread lack of access to adequately-trained health care professionals and modern medical services, or that Peruvians are failing to resort to modern health care when fatal illness strikes.

6. Living conditions vary widely by region in Peru. Lima and the other cities of the coast are better off in all respects than other areas; the rural mountain areas, and to a lesser extent the lowland jungle areas, suffer much higher rates of illness and death than the urbanized coastal areas.

7. Too many Peruvian children are suffering from communicable illnesses associated with unsanitary and impoverished living conditions, and from vaccine-preventable diseases. Peruvian public health authorities should focus their attention sharply on children living in poverty, and should press for continued and even more widespread immunization of all children against the leading immuno-preventable diseases.

8. Among specific causes of morbidity and mortality, malnutrition is discounted as a cause of illness in government records, but more than half the children in Peru under the age of six are suffering from it. Malnutrition should

be considered one of Peru's leading health problems. In addition, malaria and TBC in adults deserve greater attention due to the high social and economic impact of these diseases.

9. Relatively high morbidity generates a strong demand for curative care, and the Peruvian health sector is currently strongly oriented toward such care. Moreover, the predisposition of both medical practitioners and patients for curative rather than preventive care mitigates against a reorientation of the health services system toward a greater emphasis on preventive care, even though for the most part illness and death in Peru are preventable for other than the aged.

10. The data available in Peru on magnitude, order, differentials, structure, and trends of health status indicators at national and regional levels are reliable enough to serve as the basis for future health planning in both the primary care and hospital services areas.

Footnotes

1. This figure does not include patients discharged after normal childbirth, the main cause of hospitalizations.

2. These figures are consistent in general with those obtained by Ramos (1981) in his work on infant mortality and mother and child care in Peru.

3. However, a multivariate analysis relating these indices to outside causes is indispensable to determine more exactly the influence of health care on infant mortality.

TABLE 2.1

Population Growth, Fertility and Life Expectancy in Latin American Countries, 1980-1985

Country	Growth Rate (Per 100)	Overall Fertility Rate (Children per woman)	Life Expectancy at Birth (Years)
LATIN AMERICA	2.32	4.15	64.38
ANDEAN AREA	2.52	4.41	62.85
Bolivia	2.68	6.25	50.74
Colombia	2.14	3.93	63.63
Chile	1.68	2.90	67.01
Ecuador	3.12	6.00	62.57
Peru	**2.60**	**5.00**	**58.60**
Venezuela	3.25	4.33	67.80
ATLANTIC AREA	2.10	3.74	64.70
Argentina	1.58	3.38	69.71
Brazil	2.22	3.81	63.41
Paraguay	3.00	4.85	65.11
Uruguay	0.70	2.76	70.34
CENTRAL AMERICA MAINLAND	2.95	5.21	63.43
Costa Rica	2.63	3.50	73.03
El Salvador	2.92	5.56	64.83
Guatemala	2.91	5.17	60.72
Honduras	3.38	6.50	59.51
Nicaragua	3.32	5.94	59.81
Panama	2.17	3.46	70.98
MEXICO AND CARIBBEAN	2.37	4.36	65.49
Cuba	0.62	1.98	73.45
Haiti	2.51	5.74	52.73
Mexico	2.59	4.61	65.73
Dominican Republic	2.32	4.18	62.58

Source: CELADE 1983.

TABLE 2.2

Demographic Indicators of Peru: Observed, 1950-1980; Estimated, 1980-2005

Five-Year Period	Gross Mortality Rate (per 1000)	Infant Mortality Rate (per 1000 live births)	Life Expectancy at Birth (years)	Overall Fertility Rate (children per woman)	Gross Birth Rate (per 1000)	Growth Rate (per 1000)
OBSERVED						
1950-55	21.6	158.6	43.9	6.85	47.1	25.5
1955-60	19.7	148.2	46.3	6.85	46.8	27.1
1960-65	17.6	136.1	49.1	6.85	46.3	28.7
1965-70	15.6	126.3	51.5	6.56	43.6	28.0
1970-75	12.8	110.3	55.5	6.00	40.5	27.0
1975-80	11.7	104.9	56.9	5.38	38.0	26.3
ESTIMATED						
1980-85	10.74	98.63	58.6	5.00	36.7	26.0
1985-90	9.24	88.21	61.4	4.49	34.3	25.1
1990-95	7.69	75.81	64.6	3.97	31.2	23.5
1995-2000	6.69	66.43	67.0	3.50	28.0	21.3
2000-05	6.15	59.65	68.78	3.10	25.2	19.0

Source: INE-CELADE 1983; INE 1984a.

TABLE 2.3

Age Structure of the Peruvian Population, 1972-2000

	Age							
Year	0-5	5-14	15-24	25-44	45-64	65 & over	Total	Dependency Index
1972	16.9	26.9	18.9	22.7	11.1	3.5	100.0	91.6
1981	15.5	26.0	20.1	23.5	11.3	3.6	100.0	83.2
1986	15.1	25.1	20.2	24.4	11.6	3.6	100.0	78.8[a]
2000	12.3	23.3	19.5	27.5	13.1	4.3	100.0	66.4

a - For 1985
Sources: INE 1984a, 1985; CNP 1984b.

TABLE 2.4

Urban-Rural Population Distribution and Annual Growth Rates
Peru, 1940-2000

Year	Total population		Urban		Rural	
	Number ('000s)	Growth Rate (per 100)	%	Growth Rate (per 100)	%	Growth Rate (per 100)
1940	7,080.0		35.4		64.6	
1961	10,217.5	1.8	47.4	3.2	52.6	0.8
1972	13,954.7	2.9	59.4	5.0	40.6	0.5
1981	17,754.8	2.7	64.8	3.7	35.2	1.1
2000	27,952.1	2.0	74.6		25.4	
1940-1981		2.3		3.8		0.8

Sources: INE-CELADE 1983; INE 1984a; CNP 1984b.

TABLE 2.5

Population Distribution by Natural Regions
Peru Census, 1940, 1961, 1972, 1981

Region	1940 %	1961 %	1972 %	1981 %
Coast	28.3	39.0	46.1	50.0
Metropolitan Lima (10.4)	(18.7)	(24.4)	(27.0)	
Rest of Coast	(17.9)	(20.3)	(21.7)	(23.0)
Sierra	65.0	52.3	44.0	39.4
Jungle	6.7	8.7	9.9	10.6
Total	100.0	100.0	100.0	100.0

Source: CNP 1984.

TABLE 2.6

Demographic Conditions and Basic Sanitary Services
Peru, 1979, 1981, 1983

Department	Region (a)	Infant Mortality 1979	Life Expectancy 1983	Birth Rate 1981	Fertility Rate 1981	Mortality Rate 1983	Utilities: Water connections 1981	Utilities: Water, electricity &sew. 1981
Callao	C	54	70.8	31.2	3.4	5.5	80.3	64.4
Lima	C	56	71.0	37.5	3.6	5.6	73.2	56.4
Ica	C	66	67.7	34.7	4.7	7.1	51.8	28.3
Arequipa	S/C	68	68.0	35.3	4.6	7.1	52.7	36.0
La Libertad	S/C	73	66.7	35.0	5.2	7.7	46.8	28.4
Tacna	C	80	(36.6)	36.6	4.0	...	72.3	46.7
Moquegua	S/C	82	67.5	35.2	4.5	7.1	44.2	31.8
Tumbes	C	80	(41.0)	41.0	5.5	...	11.7	7.3
Lambayeque	C	92	(62.8)	37.5	4.9	...	49.4	31.9
Loreto	J	94	56.3	43.7	6.4	11.8	33.3	20.8
Junin	S/J	95	57.5	39.8	5.9	11.7	30.6	16.0
Madre de Dios	J	93	57.0	42.1	6.4	10.3	14.6	5.6
Cajamarca	S/J	95	55.7	41.1	7.1	13.4	11.0	7.0
San Martin	J	95	(40.7)	40.7	6.2	...	23.6	5.7
Ancash	S/C	96	(37.9)	37.9	6.1	12.7	33.8	24.9
Amazonas	J/S	96	55.3	40.6	7.4	13.0	16.1	5.0
Ucayali	J	103	43.4	43.4	6.5	...	11.9	5.3
Huanuco	S/J	107	54.9	45.1	7.0	13.5	13.0	6.4
Piura	C/S	111	42.5	42.5	6.2	...	33.1	17.8
Pasco	J/S	115	55.3	45.2	7.0	12.6	27.0	12.0
Apurimac	S	124	49.5	41.3	7.3	19.2	15.9	2.4
Puno	S	125	(38.9)	38.9	6.6	...	12.3	7.6
Ayacucho	S	120	51.0	39.6	6.9	17.3	13.6	4.9
Cuzco	S	139	47.2	42.7	6.7	19.1	22.4	9.7
Huancavelica	S	142	47.0	45.2	7.5	20.0	10.3	2.6
Average		92	60.2	37.0	5.2	10.1	41.6	28.1

Note: (a) Regions: C - Coast; S - Sierra; J - Jungle

Sources: INE 1983, 1984a, 1984b, 1985; INE-CELADE 1983; MOE 1984; CNP 1984a, 1984b.

TABLE 2.7

Rank Order by Age of Five Leading Causes of Morbidity and Mortality—Peru, 1981, 1984[a]

Causes/ Diseases[b]	<1				1-4				5-14				15-24			
	MT	MORBIDITY			MT	MORBIDITY			MT	MORBIDITY			MT	MORBIDITY		
		HD	CD	SP		HD	CD	SP		HD	CD	SP		HD	CD	SP
Perinatal	1	1														
Respiratory	2	3	1	1	1	1	1	1	1	4	1	1	3		1	1
Intestinal	3	2	2	2	2	2	2	2	3	3	2	2		5	2	2
Bacterial[c]	4		5		5		5									
Ill-def.sympt.	5				3				4				4			
Congenital		4														
Endocrine		5														
Ancyl.nec.helm.			4				4				4				5	
Viral[d]			3		4	4	3				3					
Accids.& Viol.						3		3	2	1		4	1	3		4
Other dig.tr.						5				2			5	4		
Skin								4								
Tuberculosis									5				2		4	
Upper respir.										5						
Malaria											5				3	
Dental												3				3
Abortion														2		
Neoplasms																
Dir.obstetric														1		
Fem.genitals																
Heart																
Cerebrovasc.																

a - Malnutrition should be considered among the leading causes of morbidity in children under 5 although it is not recorded as such on institutional information systems.

b - MT = Mortality (1981); HD = Hospital Discharges (1981); CD = Communicable Diseases (1984); SP = Self-Perceived (ENNSA 1984).

25-44				45-64				65 yrs+				All Ages			
MT	MORBIDITY			MT	MORBIDITY			MT	MORBIDITY			MT	MORBIDITY		
	HD	CD	SP		HD	CD	SP		HD	CD	SP		HD	CD	SP
												3			
3		1	1	3		1	1	1	5	1	1	1		1	1
		2	2			2	2			2	2	2	5	2	2
								5				4			
		5				5				5				3	
														4	
1	4				3								3		4
5	3			2	1				1				2		
															5
2		4		5		3				3					
		3				4				4				5	
			3				3								3
	2												4		
4				1	2			3	2			5			
	1												1		
	5				4										
				4	5			2	3						
								4	4						

c - Other than tuberculosis; mainly whooping cough.
d - Mainly measles in morbidity-mortality, and chicken pox in morbidity.

TABLE 2.8

Rank Order and Structure by Age of Five Leading Communicable Diseases, Peru, 1984

	Under 1		1-4		5-14		15-24		25-44		45-64		65 plus		Unident.		Total	
Diseases	Vert. %	Ord.	Vert. %	Ord.	Vert. %	Ord.	Vert. %	Ord.	Vert. %	Ord.	Vert. %	Ord.	Vert. %	Ord.	Vert. %	Ord.	Vert. %	Ord.
Acute resp.	50.22	1	43.17	1	45.35	1	38.96	1	46.68	1	50.30	1	53.29	1	28.64	2	46.12	1
Gastroent.	42.11	2	32.01	2	12.49	2	11.47	3	13.86	2	16.22	2	18.47	2	6.80	4	24.31	2
Measles	1.50	3	3.15	4													1.19	7
Helminthiasis	1.22	4	7.19	3	11.43	3	6.97	5	5.69	5	5.00	5			21.60	3	6.46	3
Influenza	1.11	5															0.22	8
Chicken pox			2.23	5	4.30	5											1.48	6
Malaria					6.22	4	11.53	2	8.47	3	5.64	4	4.04	5	29.61	1	4.08	4
Tuberculosis							8.62	4	7.84	4	7.63	3	8.91	3	4.05	5	2.62	5

Note: Vert. % = vertical, that is, calculated for all communicable diseases in the same age group
Source: OGIE 1970-84.

TABLE 2.9

Rank Order and Structure by Age of Five Leading Diagnoses of Death, Peru, 1981

Diagnosis	Under 1		1-4		5-14		15-24		25-44		45-64		65 & over		All Ages	
	Vert. %	Ord.	Vert. %	Ord.	Vert. %	Ord.	Vert %	Ord.	Vert. %	Ord.	Vert. %	Ord.	Vert. %	Ord.	Vert. %	Ord.
Perinatal	37.2	1													8.6	3
Acute respiratory	24.9	2	34.5	1	25.7	1	12.2	3	10.3	3	11.9	3	18.1	1	20.6	1
Intestinal	15.5	3	20.8	2	10.4	3									9.1	2
Other bacterial	4.5	4	6.9	5												
Ill-defined symptoms	4.1	5	8.1	3	9.3	4	6.8	4					10.8	5	8.4	4
Viral			7.4	4												
Accidents & violence					15.2	2	24.7	1	18.0	1						
Tuberculosis					5.5	5	13.2	2	12.9	2	8.6	5				
Heart											10.5	4	17.0	2		
Neoplasms									10.0	4	20.4	1	13.4	3	7.7	5
Cerebrovascular													11.7	4		
Digestive tract							5.7	5	8.0	5	12.2	2				

Note: Vert. % = calculated for all diagnoses in the same age group.
Source: OGIE 1970-84.

TABLE 2.10

Perception of Morbidity in Peru, 1984
(Rates per 100)

Variable	Total perception rate	Variable	Total perception rate
Total population	35.3		
Age:		Educational level of head of family:	
<1	63.4	Cannot read	35.9
1-4	58.8	Can read	33.5
5-14	30.5	Some high school	34.7
15-24	18.6	Some higher education	32.2
25-44	30.5		
45-64	41.0	Region:	
65 and over	51.8		
		North Coast	35.7
Sex:		Central Coast	35.4
		South Coast	26.2
Men	33.2	North Sierra	36.5
Women	37.7	Central Sierra	33.0
		South Sierra	26.4
		High Jungle	37.8
Monthly family		Low Jungle	37.8
income ('000 Soles):		Metropolitan Lima	38.9
1 - 199	40.0	Area:	
200 - 414	36.0		
415 - 800	33.2	Urban	34.6
Over 800	29.5	Rural	36.4
No information on income	33.6		

Source: ENNSA 1984.

TABLE 2.11

MOH Hospital Discharges and Length of Stay by Groups of Diagnoses, Peru, 1977, 1980

Diagnosis	1977					1980				
	Discharges			Total days	Average days	Discharges			Total days	Average days
	Number	Percent	Order			Number	Percent	Order		
Normal delivery	116,636	28.69	1	345,844	2.96	138,559	28.26	1	336,729	2.43
Direct obstetrical	25,050	6.16	4	155,302	6.19	55,307	11.28	2	435,417	7.87
Accidents & violence	33,232	8.17	2	414,615	12.47	37,543	7.66	3	613,535	16.34
Abortion	19,265	4.74	6	63,883	0.01	31,303	6.38	4	166,785	5.33
Digestive tract	27,123	6.67	3	335,228	12.35	27,386	5.59	5	561,616	15.02
Intestinal	23,715	5.83	5	199,779	3.42	26,128	5.33	6	263,748	10.09
Respiratory tract	19,240	4.73	7	205,753	10.69	24,432	4.98	7	370,690	13.94
Neoplasms	12,314	3.03	10	208,757	16.95	19,351	3.95	8	298,613	15.43
Cardio-cerebrovasc.	11,976	2.95	11	206,095	17.20	13,932	2.84	9	259,570	18.63
Tuberculosis	11,058	2.72	12	381,321	34.48	12,831	2.62	10	452,073	35.23
Female genital	15,674	3.85	8	110,243	7.03	10,400	2.12	11	108,143	10.40
Urinary tract	7,182	1.77	15	115,467	14.09	10,278	2.10	12	166,251	16.02
Ill-defined symptoms	9,565	2.35	13	89,170	9.32	8,051	1.64	13	112,235	13.94
Upper respiratory tr.	7,442	1.83	14	35,470	4.76	7,422	1.51	14	54,437	7.33
Viral	4,638	1.14	20	59,017	12.72	7,089	1.45	15	97,891	13.81
Perinatal	3,312	0.81	23	30,622	9.24	6,916	1.41	16	76,025	10.99
Musculoskeletal	5,189	1.28	18	102,050	19.67	6,480	1.32	17	150,290	23.19

(Continued)

TABLE 2.11 (Cont.)

Diagnosis	1977					1980				
	Discharges			Total days	Average days	Discharges			Total days	Average days
	Number	Percent	Order			Number	Percent	Order		
Endocrine glands	2,213	0.54	27	40,786	18.43	6,314	1.29	18	112,319	17.79
Skin	6,005	1.48	16	81,209	13.52	6,008	1.23	19	98,050	16.32
Mental disorders	5,624	1.38	17	278,409	49.50	5,892	1.20	20	524,093	88.95
Nervous system	4,694	1.15	19	106,445	22.68	4,776	0.97	21	194,033	40.63
Other bacterial	4,088	1.01	21	55,156	13.49	3,896	0.79	22	55,875	14.34
Male genital	3,352	0.82	22	49,552	14.78	3,628	0.74	23	63,773	17.58
Eye	3,225	0.79	24	32,204	9.98	3,571	0.73	24	43,001	12.04
Congenital anomalies	2,638	0.65	25	34,209	12.97	2,618	0.53	25	45,921	17.54
Blood	1,674	0.41	28	21,069	12.59	2,158	0.44	26	32,862	15.22
Other infec.& parasites	2,387	0.59	26	35,079	14.69	2,146	0.44	27	61,682	28.74
Nutritional deficiencies	15,455	3.80	9	23,838	15.43	1,720	0.35	28	35,665	20.73
Ear & mastoid	1,298	0.32	29	17,781	13.70	1,295	0.26	29	30,211	23.33
Rickets	596	0.15	30	8,251	10.84	1,153	0.24	30	18,086	15.69
Indirect obstetrical	0	0.00	33	0	0.00	716	0.15	31	6,890	9.62
Oral cavities	543	0.13	31	3,969	7.31	633	0.13	32	6,057	9.56
Venereal	190	0.05	32	2,243	11.80	392	0.08	33	4,521	11.53
Total	406,593			3,848,816	9.77	490,324			5,857,087	11.73

Source: MOH 1977-81.

TABLE 2.12

Rank Order and Structure by Age of Five Leading Diagnoses of Hospital Discharges, Peru, 1981

	Under 1		1-4		5-14		15-24		25-44		45-64		65 plus		Unident		Total	
Diagnosis	Vert. %	Ord.	Vert. %	Ord.	Vert. %	Ord.	Vert. %	Ord.	Vert. %	Ord.	Vert. %	Ord.	Vert. %	Ord.	Vert. %	Ord.	Vert. %	Ord.
Perinatal	23.28	1															1.84	9
Intestinal	23.22	2	16.05	2	10.80	3	5.76	5							9.24	3	4.87	5
Acute respiratory	16.87	3	24.79	1	9.46	4							7.30	4	8.64	4	4.08	6
Congenital	4.08	4															0.32	12
Endocrine glands	4.07	5															0.32	13
Accid. & violence			11.42	3	22.47	1	12.03	3	9.33	4	10.17	3	6.90	5	5.86	5	10.13	3
Viral			5.43	4													0.31	14
Digestive tract			4.06	5	11.46	2	8.26	4	10.66	3	20.32	1	15.53	1	10.11	2	10.61	2
Upper respiratory					6.69	5											0.49	11
Dir.obstetrical							30.16	1	26.49	1					13.79	1	16.16	1
Abortion							14.02	2	15.22	2							8.48	4
Fem.genitals									5.06	5	5.78	4					2.57	7
Neoplasms											11.90	2	11.37	2			2.41	8
Heart disease											5.25	5	10.51	3			1.47	10

Note: Vert. % = calculated for all communicable diseases in the same age group

Source: MOH 1977-81.

TABLE 2.13

Rank Order of Leading Diagnoses of Hospital Discharges by Department, Peru, 1981

Department	Obstetrical	Digest. tract	Accid. & Viol.	Abortion	Intestinal	Respiratory	Tumors	Tuberculosis	Female Genitals	Perinatal	Viral	Urinary Tract
Callao	1	2	5	3	7	4	6	-	8	-	-	-
Lima	1	2	4	3	4	7	5	-	8	-	-	-
Ica	1	3	2	5	4	6	-	7	-	8	-	-
Arequipa	1	2	5	4	3	6	-	8	-	-	-	-
La Libertad	1	2	4	3	6	5	7	9	8	-	-	-
Tacna	1	4	2	5	3	6	-	7	8	-	-	-
Moquegua	1	4	2	6	3	5	-	7	9	-	-	-
Tumbes	2	5	1	6	4	3	-	-	8	-	-	7
Lambayeque	1	4	2	5	3	6	8	-	-	7	-	-
Loreto	3	5	1	4	2	6	-	-	-	7	-	8

Junin	2	4	1	3	5	6	9	7	-	8	-	-
Madre de Dios	2	6	1	7	3	9	-	5	-	-	-	-
Cajamarca	3	2	1	5	4	6	7	-	8	-	-	-
San Martin	2	4	1	6	3	5	-	8	7	-	-	9
Ancash	1	3	2	6	4	5	-	7	-	-	-	8
Amazonas	2	3	1	7	4	5	-	6	8	-	9	-
Ucayali	1	5	2	3	4	6	-	8	7	-	-	-
Huanuco	2	5	1	6	3	4	-	8	7	-	-	-
Piura	1	2	3	5	4	6	7	-	9		-	-
Pasco	2	4	1	6	5	3	-	-	-	-	-	8
Apurimac	2	4	1	7	3	5	-	8	-	-	6	-
Puno	3	2	1	6	3	4	-	8	-	-	-	7
Ayacucho	5	4	1	6	3	2	-	7	-	-	-	8
Cuzco	2	3	1	5	4	-	6	7	-	-	-	8
Huancavelica	4	5	1	6	3	2	-	8	-	-	-	7
Total, country	1	2	3	4	5	6	7	8	-	-	-	-

Source: MOH 1977 -81.

TABLE 2.14

Infant Mortality, Life Expectancy, and Rank Order of Leading Diagnoses of Death by Department, Peru, 1981

Department	Inf. Mort. 1968	1979	Life Exp. at birth 1985	Rank order of leading diagnosis: Resp.	In-tes.	Peri-natal	Ill-def. symp.	Neopl.	Heart	Accid. and Viol.	Dig. tr.	Cere-bro-vas.	TB	Other bact.	Blood	Viral	Endo. gl.	Nerv. sys.	Nutri-tional
Callao	68	54	70.8	3	9	6	-	1	2	5	8	4	7	10	-	-	-	-	-
Lima	76	56	71.0	2	7	5	-	1	3	8	9	4	6	10	-	-	-	-	-
Ica	98	66	67.7	1	2	4	-	3	5	6	10	7	8	-	-	-	9	-	-
Arequipa	119	68	68.0	1	4	10	9	3	5	7	8	6	2	-	-	-	-	-	-
La Libertad	113	73	66.7	1	2	10	6	3	5	4	8	9	7	-	-	-	-	-	-
Tacna	111	80	(36.6)	1	3	5	10	7	6	2	8	9	4	-	-	-	-	-	-
Moquegua	130	82	67.5	1	2	4	6	-	7	3	10	8	5	9	-	-	-	-	-
Tumbes	107	88	(41.0)	1	2	3	9	10	4	6	8	5	-	7	-	-	-	-	-
Lambayeque	119	92	62.8	1	3	6	2	5	4	8	9	7	-	10	-	-	-	-	-
Loreto	131	94	56.3	1	2	5	7	3	4	9	10	8	6	-	-	-	-	-	-

Junin	153	95	57.5	1	5	2	3	6	9	4	7	-	8	-	-	-	10	-	-
Madre de Dios	149	75	57.0	3	1	7	-	-	10	2	9	-	6	-	-	4	8	-	5
Cajamarca	155	95	55.7	1	3	6	2	10	5	9	4	7	-	8	-	-	-	-	-
San Martin	126	95	(40.7)	1	2	5	4	-	8	3	-	-	-	10	6	-	9	-	7
Ancash	146	96	(37.9)	1	2	4	3	8	5	6	7	-	-	10	-	-	9	-	-
Amazonas	141	96	55.3	3	2	8	1	10	6	7	4	-	-	-	5	9	-	-	-
Ucayali	131	103	(43.4)	4	1	3	2	7	-	6	-	-	9	-	10	-	-	8	5
Huanuco	170	107	54.9	1	3	4	2	7	-	5	9	8	-	-	10	6	-	-	-
Piura	151	111	(42.5)	1	2	3	8	6	4	9	7	5	-	10	-	-	-	-	-
Pasco	168	115	55.3	1	4	2	3	10	7	5	6	-	9	-	-	8	-	-	-
Apurimac	199	124	49.5	1	4	3	2	-	9	8	6	-	-	5	-	7	10	-	-
Puno	196	125	(38.9)	1	5	3	2	-	8	7	4	-	6	10	-	-	9	-	-
Ayacucho	197	128	51.0	1	4	3	2	10	8	5	6	-	9	7	-	-	-	-	-
Cuzco	218	139	47.2	1	4	3	2	-	10	6	5	-	7	9	-	8	-	-	-
Huancavelica	227	142	47.0	1	4	2	3	-	8	6	5	-	10	9	-	7	-	-	-
Total country	142	92	60.2	1	2	3	4	5	6	7	8	9	10	11					

Source: OGIE 1975 -1981.

TABLE 2.15

Some Vaccine–Preventable Diseases Reported by Professionals in Infants Under One Year and Children From 1–4 Years
Peru, 1980-1984
(Rates per 100,000 population)

	Infants under 1 year					Children 1-4 years				
Diseases	1980	1981	1982	1983	1984	1980	1981	1982	1983	1984
Measles	413.9	282.1	362.8	206.2	334.4	389.5	186.5	242.7	137.3	260.2
Whooping Cough	278.6	292.6	203.6	165.4	172.0	180.7	161.0	107.0	94.5	93.8
Tetanus	44.6	37.3	35.1	30.5	26.0	2.7	0.5	1.5	0.7	1.3
Diphtheria	1.2	0.2	0.7	1.3	0.6	1.4	1.1	0.7	0.6	1.0
Acute Poliomyelitis	6.6	8.9	7.8	5.6	2.1	4.9	6.8	5.4	6.2	3.2
% Total Registration Coverage	61.8	69.1	72.1	73.2	75.4	61.8	69.1	72.1	73.2	75.4

Source: OGIE 1970-84.

3

Economic Crisis, Social Polarization, and Community Participation in Health Care

Judith R. Davidson and Steve Stein

Community participation in health—the involvement of low-income population segments in identifying their own health problems and helping to provide appropriate solutions—has become a central preoccupation of public health officials in many developing countries (de Kadt 1982). Implementing health care programs in which community participation (1) is actively encouraged however, has had mixed results. Community involvement in health care programs that are designed, implemented, and evaluated from outside the communities they benefit—so-called "top-down" approaches—are less successful than "bottom-up" approaches in which communities themselves design, implement, and evaluate health care programs with minimal intervention from sponsors. Peruvian communities have been increasingly involved in both "top-down" and "bottom-up" health care projects in recent years, but there has been no previous attempt to analyze the determinants of success or failure of these initiatives.

In this chapter, the responses of Peruvian communities to their health needs, and to the inadequacies of the public health sector in dealing with their health problems, are described and analyzed. After a brief discussion of the historical context of community participation in Peru, recent political, economic, and social developments affecting Peruvians' responses to their health needs are outlined. The recent emergence of a variety of community-based self-help organizations is then discussed in terms of these developments. Next, specific examples of community participation in 32 locations are summarized, and the results—both negative and positive—are analyzed. Finally, two HSA-Peru sponsored field studies of communities participating in health projects are discussed in detail. These two studies identified both top-down and bottom-up aspects of community participation, and thus serve as test cases against which the major findings of the 32 community participation projects are weighed. The chapter ends with a short summary and comments on the implications of the findings suggested by the case studies.

Sociopolitical Change and Economic Decline

Traditional Peruvian society, divided since the 16th century along ethnic and class as well as economic and political lines, was based in part on the concept of vertical, patrimonial relationships between a small, wealthy, white upper class and much larger classes of middle-income and poor *mestizos* and Indians. The former manned the country's formal institutional apparatus, ruling, exploiting, and constraining the lower classes but at the same time employing, protecting, and reassuring them. The lower classes, for their part, not only depended upon this traditional vertical structure but also supported it, even as Peru entered the period of industrialization in the 1950s and '60s. Health services, for example, were traditionally seen as the responsibility of charitable organizations created by the upper class, and more recently of the state, rather than of the medically or nutritionally needy themselves.

Toward the end of the 1960s, Peru's traditional vertical sociopolitical organization began to change. Twelve years of military rule between 1968-1980 brought further industrialization and urban population growth, and also—particularly after 1975—increasing material hardship and widespread disenchantment with the traditional order. As the effectiveness of formal institutions in ameliorating growing material pressures declined and Peru became increasingly impoverished, traditional patrimonial relationships were eroded.

In the 1970s, a series of nationalist, pro-industrial, yet interventionist economic policies were instituted by the military leadership of Peru. These were financed through foreign borrowing, resulting in a huge external debt. Combined with a sharp decline in foreign investment and rising inflation, this debt burden precipitated a profound economic crisis.

A return to democratic government under Fernando Belaunde Terry in 1980 was greeted with enthusiasm as a liberation of the state, closing an era of military government which, after 12 years in power, had lost all popular support. At first, the new President was the great civilian hope, appearing to represent a return to the benevolent patriarchy—if not the prosperity—of pre-military rule. But severe economic recession soon plagued Peru, and the new coterie of leaders appointed by Belaunde—especially those manning the political apparatus and police force—seemed remote, self-interested, and even corrupt. Belaunde himself began to be viewed by the lower classes as a traitor to popular expectations, and his incumbency did little to alleviate what had by now become a vicious circle of deepening poverty and further demoralization.

In the Belaunde years, servicing the foreign debt and implementing liberal economic policies became dominant concerns of the government. One result of these priorities was the allocation of an ever-increasing proportion of the national budget to debt service: in 1985, this commitment, along with military spending (which placed second in budgetary importance) absorbed nearly half of Peru's total government expenditures (Blacker 1985:49). Another result was a sharp rise in under- and unemployment. In 1976, 51 percent of the economically active population were fully employed, 44 percent were underemployed, and 5 percent were unemployed. In striking contrast, 1984 figures show only 32 percent fully employed, with underemployment reaching 57 percent and unemployment rising to 11 percent (Verdea 1983; Galin, Carrion and Castillo 1985).

Popular responses to this devastating combination of social polarization, economic crisis, and erosion of confidence in government probably constitute the most profound social change in modern Peruvian history (Stein and Monge 1987). Accelerating along a path first broken during the years of military rule, poor and middle-income Peruvians turned increasingly inward to their own social strata for solutions to their pressing problems, developing a variety of community-based organizations to fill the void left by the disbanding of the old hierarchical sociopolitical structure. Both destructive and constructive, these new organizations were typically informal, sometimes violence-prone, always assertively independent, and dedicated, in the long term, to the idea of a society of the masses.

In 1985, 67 percent of the electorate supported a reform-oriented coalition of a rejuvenated populist party (APRA) with the new left (Izquierda Unida). Peruvians seemed to be demanding change and reaffirming their belief in democracy at the same time. It remains to be seen whether or not the new Aprista government of Alan Garcia will incorporate representatives of the lower classes and their new kinds of community-based organizations into the Peruvian institutional apparatus. In its first year, the charismatic leadership of Garcia was at once populist and elitist, tending to impose reforms from the top down even as it promoted a philosophy of community participation.

The Informal Sector

A reflection of Peru's economic recession has been the burgeoning of the so-called "informal sector" of the urban economy. To the casual observer, informal workers appear to have taken over Lima (Carbonetto and Chavez 1984; Vargas

Llosa 1987). The most obvious are the peddlers, selling a seemingly endless variety of goods, but informals involved in certain rudimentary forms of industrial production—shoemakers, for instance, or the producers of handicrafts—are also much in evidence on the streets. Even more important in economic terms are the many who work in small-scale industry (textiles, woodworking, printing, food processing), generally on the outskirts of the city. Probably equally important are those involved in transportation and service activities: pirate taxi and bus drivers, servants, gardeners, and shoeshine boys. In Lima today, for instance, fully 95 percent of all public transportation is provided by informals (Vargas Llosa 1987). Because they are not legally employed, informals receive none of the benefits of formal employment, such as medical benefits under social security or the right to organize and press for better salaries and working conditions.

Peruvian economist Sebastian Jaure divides informal sector employment into six categories: employers (11 percent), clerical and sales employees (8 percent), manual workers (16 percent), independents, such as street vendors and messengers (58 percent), unpaid family members (7 percent), and apprentices (less than 1 percent) (Jaure 1984). There also appear to be distinct economic strata within the sector, with the employer category constituting an informal "elite," employees, workers, and apprentices forming a lower-middle level, and independents and family members—who receive the least pay and work the longest hours under the worst conditions—making up the lowest "class" of informal labor. Indeed, between half and two-thirds of those engaged in the informal sector live at a level of bare subsistence (Salcedo 1984; Grompone 1985).

Today informality forms part of Peru's most insistent contemporary dynamic: severe social polarization, which feeds on the increasingly common belief that the vertical, patrimonial relationships that have traditionally constituted the cement of post-Colonial Peruvian society are fast losing their viability. Existing formal institutions—social, religious, political and economic—seem incapable of meeting the needs of vast numbers of Peruvians, and the future offers little hope of improvement. The health status of the population and the provision of health care by those charged with that responsibility have not escaped the effects of this sociopolitical and economic crisis; one-third of the population has no access to public health services, and those services have seriously deteriorated in quality even for those largely dependent on free medical care.

Peruvian Community-Based Self-Help Organizations

In this context, many Peruvians have expressed their frustration and disillusionment in individual or collective destructiveness, from drug and alcohol abuse to terrorist activity. Many more, however, have responded to the current crisis with more constructive alternatives. They have begun to confront the problems left unaddressed after the breakdown of vertical linkages by creating new horizontal linkages among themselves. Recognizing that individual or family responses are insufficient to cope with economic and health crises, low-income Peruvians have formed hundreds of collective, grass-roots, self-help community organizations (*organizaciones de base*), to provide themselves with services only insufficiently or unreliably provided by state institutions or foreign donors. Democratic and autonomous, these organizations not only obviate the old order of vertical class relationships, but frequently challenge traditional male/female relationships as well.

In many cases, community organizations have already been highly effective. Inhabitants of *pueblos jovenes* (2), for example, are pursuing political and social goals, from legal recognition and political representation to clean water and sewage disposal systems. These communities are obligated by law to establish annually-elected councils, but in addition to such political organizations—formed either in response to government pressure or through a community's own initiative—numerous self-initiated special-interest groups have been organized to overcome deficiencies in government services or improve communities' access to services. But because of the press of other problems—safety, sanitation, nutrition, transportation—many of the poor do not place medical care at the top of their list of priorities (de Kadt 1982).

The notion of officially-supported community participation, in which local communities are persuaded to provide labor, materials, and even funding for health and other community-improvement projects designed from outside, has a long history in Latin America (de Kadt 1982). In the health care area, for example, numerous projects have incorporated the idea that communities can and should contribute manpower in the form of part-time, unpaid community health workers (CHWs). Thus in Peru, alongside the spontaneous development of self-help organizations from within communities, the government has sporadically attempted to encourage the development of similar but more formal community-based organizations, with varying degrees of success. Currently, it is the policy of the Ministry of Health (MOH) to encourage communities to participate actively and effectively in the implementation of their own health programs. But there is so much disparity in the ethnic and class composition of

Peruvian society that no single approach to encouraging this participation has been found to be effective across communities.

There are three methods by which community participation in health programs can be achieved. *Resources mobilization*, based on a "top-down" health care delivery ideology, assumes that the primary obligation of a community toward the management of its health care is to supply materials and labor. Community participation through mobilization begins outside the community; the planning, implementation, and evaluation of health projects are the responsibility of the formal health sector, represented by MOH or private voluntary organization (PVO) personnel. A second method, the *intervention* of the MOH or PVOs in the development of primary health services, can be the product of either a "top-down" or a "bottom-up" health delivery ideology; community members are more actively engaged in planning, implementation, and evaluation than under the mobilization ideology, but training programs and organizing activities are still initiated from outside beneficiary communities. A third method, the *self-direction* of health projects, in contrast, exemplifies a "bottom-up" ideology: the thrust of action lies not outside communities but within them. Self-direction can occur in response to a health delivery system brought into a community from outside, but it is implemented by independent *organizaciones de base* with minimal outside assistance.

Two examples of contemporary autonomous popular action are illustrative: communal kitchens and glass-of-milk programs. Both are responses to malnutrition, a basic fact of life in urban as well as rural Peru and a direct result of the poverty brought on by Peru's twin sociopolitical and economic crises. Malnutrition is becoming more rather than less prevalent in Peru; in 1979, 70 percent of Lima's population was critically malnourished, and given the fact that real income has fallen since then, the present number of undernourished Limans has reached appalling proportions (Grados *et al.* 1980; Vilchez 1983).

The proliferation of communal kitchens in Lima's *pueblos jovenes* is a palpable instance of community response to the failure of the state to answer the needs of the urban poor. These organizations lower the cost of feeding families, generally by receiving donations of food and in some cases by buying food in quantity. Costs are also reduced by the adoption of production-line techniques of food preparation. Previously prepared food is taken from communal kitchens into individual homes, where it typically provides the major daily meal for all family members (Sara-Lafosse 1984).

Obtaining milk, a major source of protein for children, is particularly difficult because of its expense; in 1984, for example, a liter of milk cost 960 *soles*, but the poorest families in one squatter settlement in Lima earned a daily average income of only 884 *soles* per person (Vieira 1984). Tea often replaces milk in the bottles of infants to momentarily assuage their hunger. In response to this situation, mothers have formed numerous glass-of-milk (*vaso de leche*) committees, which purchase and distribute dried milk powder and other nutritional supplements and flavoring agents (sugar, cinnamon, anise) to young children and expectant mothers. The costs of these ingredients are covered by small weekly contributions from participating families. By buying milk in powdered form and in bulk, the *vaso de leche* committees can provide beneficiaries with more nutrition at less expense.

Analysis of Community Participation Projects

Methodology

The variety and extent of Peruvian community participation in the specific area of health care was assessed under the HSA-Peru in a study of 32 health projects, implemented both in urban *pueblos jovenes* and in rural communities (Table 3.1). The latter represented a wide range of ecological, geographical, and social-structural settings, including traditional Indian communities of the southern highlands, tribal villages of the Amazon jungle, and agricultural cooperatives and mining communities in the north. Sponsors included national PVOs with ties to international funding agencies, national PVOs without such ties, and international development agencies implementing joint projects with the MOH. All of the projects had multiple aims, which included the training of community health workers such as traditional birth attendants or health promoters, the formation of community organizations such as glass-of-milk committees, census-taking, immunization campaigns, fund-raising, and the implementation of preventive health projects such as latrine construction.

For each project, data on a set of ten variables were collected, including the project's goals, activities, and achievements; obstacles to full community participation; and the ecological, economic and sociopolitical characteristics of the community. All health activities (for example, the construction of health facilities, the training of CHWs, community census-taking, the identification of tuberculosis patients) were identified and categorized into one of 20 types, and their means of implementation—resources mobilization, intervention, or self-direction—described (HSA-Peru 1986d:App.III). In the 32 projects studied (each of which had attempted multiple activities), very few specific activities had been successfully implemented through mobilization (only 14); successes were much more often accomplished through intervention (120) or self-direction (121).

Overall Results

In 25 of the 32 projects reviewed, actual achievements fell short of objectives. This is hardly surprising, since most of the organizations reviewed had planned combinations of short- and long-range objectives; at any given point in time, certain activities had been completed while others had only begun. There was, however, a patterned relationship between the objectives of sponsors and their achievements—one that was correlated with different communities' varying ecological, sociocultural, sociopolitical and economic characteristics. Communities with a long history of struggles with the establishment, for example, were more apt to produce strong community organizations that provided a basis for the development of health activities. Only some of the organizations sponsoring the 32 projects had taken these structural characteristics into account when setting goals for their programs; many appeared not to recognize the important role played by such variables.

These 32 cases highlighted the significant differences between urban settlements and rural communities in Peru. Generally speaking, the absence of services and of traditional social structures in both *pueblos jovenes* and urban sqatter settlements creates vacuums that residents and outside agencies seek to fill, often complementing each other in the process. In rural communities, on the other hand, static organizational structures, reinforced by cultural and economic conditions, may provide resistance to penetration by the formal health system.

Perhaps the most widely-recognized national attempt at implementing a health program through community participation in Peru has been the massive training of CHWs—mainly traditional birth attendants and health promoters. An elemental part of such training is the establishment and operation of local "health committees," whose primary goal is to activate programs set up by PVOs or MOH regional planners and administrators, in response to national health directives. Under ideal conditions, health committees function as the means through which community resource mobilization occurs, decisions about training operations are made, and training programs are instituted. On the whole, however, the health committee concept has been difficult to implement successfully.

Obstacles to Community Participation

Some of the many obstacles to full participation in community health projects that were identified by the case study review were rooted within communities. In other instances, the lack of success seems to have been a product of externally-imposed rather than internally-existing problems.

One particularly important internal obstacle to community participation was the pre-existing internal hierarchy of a community. Efforts to establish community-based health care were much less apt to be successful when they were undertaken without regard for indigenous sociopolitical organization. It is clearly not enough merely to understand the pattern of local leadership; equally important is an appreciation of the power structure that dictates relationships between social or hereditary groups. A second commonly-encountered internal obstacle was conflicts within a community. If, for example, there is strong factionalism in a community, programs that involve the members of one faction may offend the members of others. Third, the lack of prior political activism appeared to be an important internal determinant of the extent to which communities will achieve full participation. Fourth, the isolation of some rural communities sometimes made it difficult to find CHWs. Finally, the non-utilization of health programs or non-compliance of patients with providers seemed to stem from dissonance between the modern medical model followed by health program sponsors and the traditional one understood by community members. Some underlying causes of this problem are a lack of a mutual understanding between provider and patient about illness etiology, physiological principles, or the effects of western vs. traditional drugs; a lack of respect for or knowledge of the functions of traditional health care providers; and lack of understanding of the expected roles of provider and patient.

External obstacles to success most frequently centered on the MOH—particularly on its community-based health teams and CHW training program. The behavior and attitudes of MOH-trained health workers, whether community members or outsiders, caused frequent problems. In some cases community members perceived a lack of sensitivity on the part of MOH physicians, nurses, and other health care providers to their needs; in others, they felt the visits of MOH personnel were irregular or infrequent, that personnel moved too frequently from community to community, or that input from community members was sometimes ignored in the design and evaluation of health programs or the establishment of native health committees according to MOH criteria (3). Sometimes the health resources provided by the MOH were viewed as insufficient. Finally, the attentions of indigenous health promoters were often seen as focused on income-producing (*e.g.*, selling medicines) rather than the health services they were paid to administer, while their true allegiance was to the MOH rather than to their communities.

Field Studies

Based on a review of the 32 projects described above, field studies in two *pueblos jovenes* in Lima with ongoing health care projects involving community participation were designed under HSA-Peru auspices and carried out through the private Peruvian research group DESCO, under the direction of Peruvian sociologist Luis Olivera Cardenas (see Olivera Cardenas 1986). These two studies represented a test of the general findings of the earlier 32-case review, and more specifically of the variables that had been identified as determining the nature of community participation.

The two settlements studied illustrate some of the historical, cultural, and political complexities involved in carrying out health projects in Peru. Both are located in the huge San Juan Miraflores (SJM) district of Lima, where 70 percent of residents live in substandard housing and suffer from impoverished living conditions. Ongoing health care projects involving community participation have been implemented in both. But the two communities are quite different in the number of years of their existence, in the extent and type of their internal organization, and in their linkages with the formal health care system.

The SJM District, composed of many different settlements, has two health centers, 19 health posts, and a total of 99 community organizations concerned with health issues on a continuous basis. These include health promoter committees (working under the umbrella of the two health care facilities), numerous glass-of-milk committees, a maternity center, and a tuberculosis patients' program. Some of these community organizations are genuine, grass-roots community organizations, while others reflect the efforts of the MOH or PVOs to foster community participation in health.

The first field study took place in the Virgen del Buen Paso (VBP) settlement, one of the oldest *pueblos jovenes* in Lima and home to some 400 families—many of them still without permanent housing. This twenty-year-old community had had an early history of activism. In 1965, when the settlers first arrived, they were removed from the area in which they originally camped and relocated in the zone they now occupy. Subsequently, motivated by the urgent need for housing, community members created a settlers' organization that worked actively to achieve permanent residency. In 1972, however, government officials decided that a new organization, based on a vertical model, should assume leadership in VBP. The autonomy toward which the community had been working was thus eroded, and its objective of constructing a social base from which to support local actions was defeated. The settlers' organization continued in existence, but without its former dynamism. Even the eventual dismantling of the vertical organization, in 1977, failed to revive it.

During the 1960s and 1970s, foreign aid organizations entered many communities like VBP, separately implementing their aid plans from the outside. This intervention may have given rise to the conformist and passive behavior that still characterizes some settlements—a hypothesis that the VBP case supports. Since the late 1970s, many of these organizations have redefined the methods according to which they deliver their services to communities, but by that time the VBP population had become accustomed to outside organizations of this type solving their problems.

VBP has a health post—part of a MOH-UNICEF assistance plan—that was built in 1983-84 with construction materials provided by UNICEF and labor provided by the community. This was a typical "top-down" effort, illustrating the resources mobilization approach to community participation. The facility now has its own permanent medical staff, paid by the MOH, consisting of a doctor and a trained midwife who attend twice weekly, plus a dentist and psychologist (once a week). These physical and human resources notwithstanding, the VBP health post lacks the necessary equipment, personnel, and supplies to cover basic disease prevention and sanitary education in the community.

In addition to its medical personnel, the health post has a team of health promoters drawn from the VBP population. These CHWs, trained under the MOH-UNICEF agreement and now in charge administering the facility six days a week, were selected without regard to the sociopolitical organization of the community. Moreover, decisions regarding the health post are not made by the population it serves. Thus the health promoters are not closely involved with the community; they keep their distance, remaining autonomous and self-sufficient, out of tune with the perceived needs of the community. Several of them carry out administrative functions rather than providing primary health care, and their number has declined due to failure to appoint replacements. According to the head of the VBP health promoter team, the community is accustomed to having people come in from outside to tell them what to do. Thus the team feels it must frequently call on outside practitioners, who—although they may know nothing about the reality of the peoples' lives and problems—are listened to more than than the health promoters.

VBP also has a glass-of-milk committee, which has enjoyed somewhat greater success than the health promoter program and illustrates a bottom-up, "self-directed" kind of community participation. It is organized by residential blocks, with a coordinator, elected by the beneficiary families on each block, responsible for collecting and distributing milk that arrives from the SJM District Council. A general coordinator oversees the program, but the actual distribution of dried milk—a daily task—rests on a dynamic and efficient organization of mothers, who meet regularly to discuss the details of milk distribution and to monitor and evaluate the operation of the program. A permanent mechanism for communication among neighbors has thus been created. There is considerable interest on the part of the women of VBP—especially the mothers—in trying to solve the problem of malnutrition among the community's children, and the women's initiative in the glass-of-milk program opens up the possibility of extending their work to other health-related areas, such as immunization campaigns. However, the organizational experience of the glass-of-milk committee is not integrated with the overall health activities carried out within the community.

The second community studied by DESCO was Sarita Colonia (SC), a relatively new settlement in SJM composed primarily of young, second-generation migrant families with an urgent need for housing. This community lacks both running water and electricity; trucks carry water to the entrance of the settlement so that residents can carry it to their homes, and electricity is brought clandestinely into the community by tapping lines in neighboring settlements. But despite this poverty, the community's five residential blocks are well organized; in each one, a popularly elected director coordinates with the central directive board. The community's strong leaders, about whom there has grown up a certain popular mystique, recognize the need for organization, for community participation in decision-making, and for creating channels for the people to express themselves democratically.

The main concern of the SC community has been to obtain legal recognition, and to that end the central directive board has contracted private engineers at considerable expense, has had the necessary plans drawn up, and is now negotiating to obtain legal and official recognition. Meanwhile, attention to health problems has been left largely to the women of the community as a secondary concern. The community receives no services from the MOH, but there is a grass-roots glass-of-milk committee, benefitting 168 children, which was organized by community mothers to help fight malnutrition. The cost of necessary ingredients for the program is covered by a weekly contribution from each family amounting to 300 *soles* An assembly consisting of all the program's adult participants meets every 15 days to elect (rotating) coordinators and to discuss the organization of work shifts, the amount of weekly payments, and future activities (including health activities).

Among the women of Sarita Colonia there is a high degree of participation in the glass-of-milk program ("for our children, no effort is too much"). The program also satisfies the women's desires to better themselves by learning, socializing, and exchanging views with others. It is important to note the extent to which this program serves as a means for promoting and developing community solidarity: organizing work shifts, deciding how to distribute among members the costs of the quota when someone is too poor to pay, and discussing the care of abandoned children, old people, or tuberculosis victims are strongly unifying activities.

The glass-of-milk committee in SC now enjoys a position in the community from which other activities, such as promoting health care and setting up a communal dining room, can be carried out. In the summer of 1985, for example, the committee implemented campaigns, promoted by both the provincial and district municipalities, to combat diarrhea and dehydration in children, and mothers were trained in the use of packaged rehydration salts. The successful implementation of this project suggests the great potential of the collective involvement of women in community health projects. More generally, the mechanisms of community participation at work in Sarita Colonia illustrate the successful implementation of initiatives coming up from below, and thus promoting the active involvement of a large segment of the population.

The Virgen del Buen Paso and Sarita Colonia case studies illustrate, in very different ways, the potential impact of community-based health organizations in Peru. In VBP, the "top-down" way in which the health promoter project organizers have worked has discouraged the population's participation. The role played by the MOH, which operates the health post, is very formal, and its relationship with the population is vertical: the MOH provides training and professional services in the health post, while the population, which contributed its labor to the construction of the facility, remains outside the decision-making process. Community participation is sought through a structure imposed from outside and with objectives defined by outsiders.

The VBP community has a history of receiving assistance, and is organizationally weak. Its health promoter committee has not been greatly concerned with the organization and cohesion of the population. It has shown little interest in health problems except for the installation and operation of the health post; once that was functioning, it withdrew from operational aspects, thus tacitly accepting the vertical relationship between the public health system and the population. Community leaders demand that new promoters be trained, but do not call upon them to accept an outreach role in health promotion except to make sure that the management of the health posts remains in reliable hands. And because of its vertical relationship with the community, the health promoter committee does not appear to its members as representing their interests. In fact, a differentiation in prestige has arisen, with promoters now viewed as better-trained than other community members and of higher status because they represent a governmental entity. Despite the fact that similar health promoter committees exist in several settlements in the district, these groups have no common form and remain isolated from one another; consequently, there is no opportunity to share experiences.

In VBP, community participation in health care has been limited to the promoter group itself, excluding the rest of the population. And since the committee's involvement in community affairs has been solely through the health post and its administration, planning and assessment have remained outside the committee; it has no role in decisions such as those concerning personnel or resources. Its work style has strengthened the vertical scheme, which has discouraged community involvement to the extent that community members now see their participation as embodied in the neighborhood organization that represents them.

Yet new forms of participation have emerged in VBP in recent years, exemplified by the glass-of-milk committee. These organizations, characterized by horizontal relationships and joint action, have opened up new forms of relationships and have suggested new ways to face problems. This kind of experience has not yet become widespread enough in the settlement for the overall vertical relations between the population and external powers to be questioned. However, horizontal organizational structures do exist, and the present vertical community structure could change toward a horizontal and more democratic one as a result.

In the case of Sarita Colonia, we find relationships among some residents that bode well for the development of further community participation. In the glass-of-milk program, the basis of action came from the population itself, which set up its own organization to face its own malnutrition problems. Due solely to the community's initiative, an autonomous mechanism of participation developed without the imposition of influence from any outside agency. The SC glass-of-milk committee's work involves the mothers in the settlement; it depends on their support and on the community's recognition of their work. The committee is a vital organization, managing daily operations that by their very nature guarantee permanent service to the population. Establishing a stable network of women, cementing their solidarity and autonomy, and training them to run their operations themselves are among the principal achievements of this organization.

The internal organization of SC has encouraged the involvement of the entire population in resolving urgent problems. Community members have managed to establish permanent, democratic mechanisms for action, such as decision-making assemblies of all the people. Because of the community's overriding concern with legal recognition, health problems do not yet receive sufficient attention in SC. However, the glass-of-milk committee's success, and its larger concern with nutrition and health, hint that the community will soon be making these matters a higher priority.

By comparing the two field studies, one can better appreciate the specific points that differentiate the different "models" of participation. In the case of Virgen del Buen Paso, we have an organization based on outside initiative, with bureaucratic relationships among its members and between it and the population—an organization that lacks a clear vision of its role in the future of the community and of its place among the rest of the community's organizations. In Sarita Colonia, on the other hand, we have an organization that has arisen as a result of a population's own initiative, one that enjoys dynamic relationships among its own members and with the general population—relationships that are expressed in joint projects involving the whole community.

These two communities are in different stages of their development. It may be that the energy and activism that characterized the VBP settlement in its early years was blunted and dissipated by interaction with the government and other outside agencies. If so, it remains to be seen whether or not the youthful dynamism and widespread community participation of SC will be reduced to dependence by the same forces. On the other hand, SC may be coming of age in a period in which more support for community self-direction is available.

Conclusions

Summary

From the colonial period through the mid-twentieth century, due to a variety of political, social, economic and cultural factors, poor and middle-class Peruvians historically tended to look up the sociopolitical hierarchy, rather than to themselves, for direction and help in health care. Since the 1970s, however, with the onset of a profound crisis in Peru producing extreme levels of social polarization, there has been growing disenchantment with an increasingly ineffective system of traditional helping mechanisms and institutions, and a concomitant tendency—if only a tendency, at this point—for communities to turn inward for answers to social problems, such as malnutrition and inadequate health care. Recently—particularly in urban *pueblos jovenes*—grass-roots, community-based self-help organizations have emerged, which have to an extent filled gaps left by the disintegration of the old hierarchical structure.

Prior to the HSA-Peru, Peruvian experiences with health care projects involving the active participation of community members had not been systematically reviewed, nor had the important lessons inherent in these experiences been identified. Thirty-two such projects for which records of activities had been methodically kept, representing a great variety of cultural and ecological settings as well as degrees of success or failure, were analyzed. Each had been implemented under one of three different ideologies: resources mobilization, a "top-down" approach in which communities provide resources and sponsors provide inspiration, implementation, direction and evaluation; intervention, in which outside authorities intervene in communities to the limited extent of organizing projects and training community members to carry them out; or self-direction, in which communities perceive the responsibility for their health care as being their own, and—even if they must rely on outside resources—implement self-help programs accordingly.

Two major conclusions emerged from a review of the 32 cases. First, because of the wide variety among Peruvian communities, no single, uniform approach to fostering community participation in health care can be effective everywhere;

rigidly-planned programs that provide little consideration of local cultural, social, or political variables often meet with considerable community resistance. Second, programs implemented under the resources mobilization ideology not only fail to alleviate the problem of the dependence and passivity of rural and semi-urban populations—they actually contribute to it; and, conversely, self-directed programs reduce the historical passive/dependent tendencies of Peruvian communities. Effective community participation simply cannot be imposed from above; it must arise from within a community.

The study also suggested that community participation projects initiated and directed by the Ministry of Health have been less successful, in general, than those implemented by private voluntary organizations (4). The health promoter concept, especially, has been fraught with problems; within their communities, health promoters are viewed as having been selected by the MOH rather than by community members, but—though trained in MOH programs—they are not considered by the MOH to be part of its health personnel hierarchy. Community health committees that in many cases have been organized on MOH insistence, as a way of stimulating community participation, have been superimposed on existing community leadership organizations that subsequently refuse to cooperate with them. The MOH has also been criticized for failing to deliver health services and medicines on a regular basis once a primary health care program has been initiated.

The review also showed that the most effective, self- directed community participation in health care in Peru exists in urban rather than rural communities—a finding that may reflect the prior experiences of the urban poor in organizing themselves for common goals.

A number of factors, both internal and external, influence community participation in health care. Of the internal factors, a community's ability to organize itself, the amount of priority it gives to health, and its prior organizational activity appear to be among the most important. Significant external factors include the policy orientation of the sponsor (whether the MOH or any other organization) and the community's degree of dependence on MOH or PVO leadership and resources.

To field-test some of the lessons learned from the 32 case studies, a thorough examination of the extent and variety of community participation in health care in two *pueblos jovenes* in Lima was undertaken. In general, the results of this exercise supported the most significant conclusions of the earlier review of cases—that a "bottom-up" implementation of projects is more successful than a "top-down" approach to community participation, and that in order for projects to achieve their goals sponsoring organizations must take the pre-existing organizational structure of communities into account.

Implications of Findings

Together, the 34 case studies make clear the vital importance of understanding social and ethnic distinctions between Peruvians and their long-established communal structures and systems, and of permitting communities a generous hand in designing, implementing, and evaluating their own health care programs. While these basic observations represent the best-substantiated and most important findings of the case studies, a number of other observations, with implications for future public health care policy, also emerged.

1. The Peruvian health delivery system is still overly dependent upon sponsoring agencies.

2. The reason why PVOs seem to be more successful than government health agencies at sponsoring projects that make use of the internal structures of existing community organizations (or encourage their development) may be that PVOs tend to target specific communities or specific problems, and can thus tailor their projects to particular requirements and circumstances. It may also be because their projects are smaller and more focused; they can thus accomplish better community analysis and needs assessment before designing their projects. Then, too, successfully encouraging community self-direction may at times have unforeseen political repercussions, which may be less threatening to private than to government organizations.

3. The appropriate mechanisms for successful community participation in health activities vary according to the history, culture, economy, and ecology of different communities, but government agencies, obliged to make and carry out health policy on a nationwide scale, are often ill-equipped to take the diversity of their huge catchment areas into account.

4. The success of some sponsoring organizations in initiating community participation that becomes an integral part of the internal structure of a community is evidence that this is an achievable goal. Reform-oriented sponsoring organizations can motivate communities to take leadership of and responsibility for their health programs, by assuring that community members participate in all phases of program development.

5. Community participation in health programs is an important element in the new structure of the health sector under the Garcia government. Communities are expected to identify their health needs themselves, to develop primary health care services appropriate to meeting those needs, and to demand outside support from the state at the department level. In continuing to implement "top-down" health care programs, however, the new government's behavior is at odds with its own policy.

Footnotes

1. In its broadest sense, the term "community participation" suggests the direct involvement of community members in the decisions and actions that affect their lives. In actual practice, it may suggest a whole range of behaviors, from the mobilization of community resources to increased control on the part of community leaders over the social, political, economic, and environmental factors that affect their constituencies. While these alternate views of participation are not necessarily incompatible, they do reflect different foci of social analysis—especially with respect to the distribution of wealth and power among different social groups (Muller 1983).

2. Recently-settled, low-income communities, usually located at the margins of urban areas, on land made available for settlement by the government.

3. The only local input permitted by MOH regulations is the selection of members.

4. While there have been training programs initiated by non-governmental sponsoring organizations that stress community independence, these have not been objectively evaluated, so it is difficult to comment on possible differences in the outcome of programs initiated by governmental vs. non-governmental sponsors.

TABLE 3.1

Sponsoring Organizations for Health Projects Involving Community Participation

Sponsoring Organizations	Project Locations/ Health Region	Source of Data
1. Save the Children; UNICEF; Comunidad Cristiana; Universidad de San Marcos; Ministerio de Salud; CEPROC (Centro de Promocion Comunal); CESPAC; CIDIAG; Manuela Ramos; CCPVS (Centro de Comunicacion Popular de Villa el Salvador); Calandria (Asociacion de Comunicadores Sociales)	Villa El Salvador (Lima/Callao)	Document: Informe General de Actividades del Consejo de Salud de la Cuaves a la V Convencion, Villa el Salvador, Julio de 1985. CUAVES (ms.)
2. CARE	Collique (Lima/Callao)	Document: Aproximacion Diagnostica de un Sector de Collique IV, Zona, Mayo 1985. CARE (ms.)
3. ASI (Asociacion para la Salud Integral)	La Providencia; 15 de Enero; Sagrado Modero; Maria Auxiliadora; Canto Chico; Nuevo Peru; San Milarion (Lima/Callao)	Interviews: Oscar Lazarte, M.D. (Director) 105 Las Paiques 655, Coop. Las Flores, San Juan Lurigancho

(Continued)

TABLE 3.1 (Cont.)

Sponsoring Organizations	Project Locations/ Health Region	Source of Data
4. ALTERNATIVA (Centro de Educacion y Capacitacion Popular)	Puente Piedra; San Martin de Porras (Lima/Callao)	Interviews: Bruno Benavides, M.D. Emeterio Perez 348 Urbanizacion Ingenieria
5 INSAP (Instituto de Salud Popular)	Villa Vitarta; Manylsa (Lima/Callao)	Interviews: Arturo Iglesias B., M.D. (Director) Av. Arsenales 1080-303
6. CAAP (Centro Amazonico Antropologia y Aplicacion)	San Martin (Chiclayo)*	Interviews: Clemencia Arambura/ Rosa Sveiro (Antropologas) Av. Gonzales Prada 626, Magdelena
7. CELATS (Centro Latinoamericano de Trabajo Social)	Villa Venturo; Chorrillos (Lima/Callao)	Document: Proyecto de Educacion Popular en Salud Para la Comunidad de Villa Venturo (ms.) Interviews: project coordinators
8. IAC (Instituto Andino Culturales)	Canete-Mala (Lima/Callao)	Interviews: Judy Hamje (enfermera) Pumacawa 1364, Jesus Maria
9. CICDA (Centro Internacional de Cooperacion para el Desarrollo Agricola)	Chumbivilca-Cusco (Cusco)	Document: La Salud en CICDA. Rastreo de una Evolucion a Traves de la Documentacion Interna. Pierre de Zutter, Lima, 1985

10. CICDA (Centro Internacional de Cooperacion para el Desarrollo Agricola)	La Union-Arequipa (Arequipa)	Document: La Salud en CICDA. Rastreo de una Evolucion a Traves de la Documentacion Interna. Pierre de Zutter, Lima, 1985
11. Centro Flora Tristan	San Juan de Lurigancho (Lima/Callao)	Document: Child Care in Urban and Rural Peru: A Report Presented to the Overseas Education Fund of the League of Women Voters. Jeanine Anderson, Lima, June 1979 (ms.) Interview: Nancy Palomino (profesora) Parque Hernan Velarde, #42, Lima
12. Programa de Salud de Villa Ventura	Villa Ventura (Lima/Callao)	Published article: Exposicion Villa Ventura. *Cuaderno Celats* 32: 23-35. Equipo de Profesionales, 1981
13. Equipo Multidisciplinario de Salud	Cono Norte-Lima (Lima/Callao)	Published article: Exposicion Equipo Multi-disciplinario Cono Norte, Lima. *Cuaderno Celats* 32: 35-41. Equipo Multidisciplinario de Salud, 1981
14. CIDESCA (Consejo Integrado para el Desarrollo Campesina)	Chancay (Chiclayo)*	Published article: Exposicion Consejo Integrado para el Desarrollo Campesino-Chiclayo. *Cuaderno Celats* 32:65-77. CIDESCA, 1981
15. Centro de Educacion Familiar	Chimbote (Trujillo)	Published article: Exposicion de Centro de Educacion Familiar. *Cuaderno Celats* 32:59-65. Centro de Educacion Familiar, 1981

(Continued)

TABLE 3.1 (Cont.)

Sponsoring Organizations	Project Locations/ Health Region	Source of Data
16. CITUP (Comite de Investigacion y Trabajo Universitario Popular)	Arequipa (Arequipa)	Published article: Informe del Comite de Investigacion y Trabajo Universitario Popular (CITUP) sobre la Experiencia Piloto en el Pueblo Joven Augusto Freyere Garcia Monterroso 1976-1980. *Cuaderno Celats* 32:77-89. CITUP, 1981
17. CFC (Centro de Formacion Campesina)	Sicuani; Yanoaca (Cusco)	Published article: Exposicion C.F.C., Cusco. *Cuaderno Celats* 32: 89-101. C.F.C., 1981
18. DESCO (Centro de Estudios de Promocion y Desarrollo)	Huancavelica (Ica); Huaral (Lima); Purisima; Congas (Trujillo) San Juan de Luriguancho; Nuevo Peru; Maria Auxiliadora; Canto Chico; Sagrado Madero (Lima)	Published article El Trabajo de Promocion en Proyectos de Salud, La Experiencia de DESCO. Miguel Saravia. In *Experiencias de Desarrollo Popular en el Campo de la Medicina Tradicional y Moderna*, edited by Luis Miguel Saravia C. and Rosa Suiero Cabredo. Lima, CAAP/DESCO, 1985
19. PNUD, OPS	Alto Amazonas; Maranon; Ucayali; Bajo Amazonas; Napo (Chiclayo)*	Published article: Proyectos de Desarrollo y y Extension de Servicios de Salud en la Region de Loreto. Rosario Torres Bazan. In *Experiencias de Desarrollo Popular en el Campo de la Medicina*

		Tradicional y Moderna, edited by Luis Miguel Saravia C. and Rosa Suiero Cabredo. Lima, CAAP/DESCO, 1985
20. CICDA (Centro Internacional de Cooperacion para el Desarrollo Agricola)	(Cusco; Arequipa)	Published article: Actitud de los Proyectos Frente a la Medicina Moderna y a la Medicina Tradicional. CICDA. In *Experiencia de Desarrollo Popular en el Campo de la Medicina Tradicional y Moderna*, edited by Luis Miguel Saravia C. and Rosa Suiero Cabredo. Lima, CAAP/DESCO, 1985
21. PIHUAN	(Cajamarca)	Published article: Formacion y Capacitacion de Promotores de Salud. Groupo PIHUAN. In *Experiencia de Desarrollo Popular en el Campo de la Medicina Tradicional y Moderna*, edited by Luis Miguel Saravia C. and Rosa Sueiro Cabredo. Lima, CAAP/DESCO, 1985
22. CIDESCA	Chiclayo (Chiclayo)*	Published article: Capacitacion a Promotores de Salud 77-81, Chiclayo. *Cuadernos Celats* 37: 31-37. CIDESCA, 1982
23. Swiss Government/UNICEF	(Puno)	Document: Evaluacion del Proyecto Extension de la Atencion Medica Rural en el Peru, October 1980. Swiss Government Technical Cooperation, ORDEPUNO Region and MOH, 1980

(Continued)

TABLE 3.1 (Cont.)

Sponsoring Organizations	Project Locations/ Health Region	Source of Data
24. Puno Regional Development Board	(Puno)	Published article: From the Child to Community Participation: Lessons from Two Peruvian Experiences. Manuel Tejada Cano. *Assignment Children* 47/48, 1979
25. CEDAP (Centro de Desarrollo Agropecuario)	(Ayacucho)	Published article: Hacia un Trabajo de Salud en Comunidades Campesinas de Ayacucho. *Cuadernos Celats* 37: 17-23. CEDAP, 1982
26. GTZ/MOH (Sociedad Alemna de Cooperacion Tecnica and the Peruvian Ministry of Health)	(Cusco)	Published report: Proyecto de Atencion Primaria y Desarrollo de Servicios de Salud de Cusco, Apurimac, y Madre de Dios, Tomo I-III, Cusco. Peruvian Ministry of Health, 1982
27. Proyecto Servicios Integrados de Salud y Generacion de Ingresos Para las Familias del Valle del Chillon	Chillon; Rimac; Lurin (Lima)	Internal documents
28. Equipo Socio-Sanitario	(Cusco)	Published article: Actitud de los Proyectos Frente a la Medicina Moderna y a la Medicina Tradicional. Diana de Tomaso, Andrea Caprara, and Edoardo Chiesa. In *Experiencias de Desarrollo*

		Popular en el Campo de la Medicina Tradicional y Moderna, edited by Luis Miguel Saravia C. and Rosa Sueiro Cabrado. Lima, CAAP/DESCO, 1985
29. AID/MOH Promoter Training Program	National (Trujillo)	Unpublished evaluation report: Evaluation, Health Promoter Program, Ministry of Health, Peru, January–June 1984, Volumes 1 and 2. Boston, Management Sciences for Health, 1984
30. Equipo de Salud de la Granja Escuela "Pumamarka" de Yucay, Cusco	(Cusco)	Report: Servicio de Promocion de Salud y Atencion Primaria en las Comunidades Campesinas de las Provincias de Calca y Urubamba (ms.). Santiago Saco, Carmen Valeocia, and B. Yolanda Zambrano. August, 1982
31. Universidad Cayetano Heredia	(Lima)	Report: Organizacion de Delegados de Salud en el Pueblo San Juan de Dios 5to. Sector Ermitano Alto-Distrito de Independencia (ms.) Flor Vasquez Galvez and Jorge Silva Leguia. Lima, 1982
32. CCAIJO (Centro de Capacitacion Agro Industrial Jesus Obrero)	Occuran; Pinchimuru; Pampaccamara; (Cusco)	Book: *Participacion Popular en Programas de Atencion Sanitaria Primaria en America Latina.* Frederick Muller. Medellin, Universidad de Antioquia Facultad Nacional de Salud Publica, 1979

*Note: Chiclayo is the Lambayeque—Amazonas region

4

Private Health Care Financing Alternatives[1]

Julio Castañeda Costa and José Carlos Vera la Torre

The contemporary Peruvian health care delivery system, characterized in Chapter 1 as a mixture of private and public providers and unevenly-distributed physical and human resources, covers the Peruvian population only incompletely. To review: the *Ministry of Health* (MOH), funded from general taxes and foreign donor support, administers 59 percent of the hospital beds, accounts for 27 percent of the country's total health care expenditures, and provides access to its health services for approximately 26 percent of the population (see also Ch. 8). The *Social Security Institute* (IPSS), funded from wage taxes, operates 15 percent of the hospital beds yet is responsible for 33 percent of all health care expenditures; it is legally mandated to cover about 18 percent of the population, but provides access to its services for only about 13 to 14 percent (see also Ch. 9). *The private sector*, supported by direct household and third-party (insurance) payments, administers only 18 percent of the hospital beds yet accounts for 34 percent of total health care expenditures, and provides coverage to 21 percent of the population.

This leaves an estimated 32 percent of the population—who are at the bottom of the socioeconomic ladder—without access to modern health services. Part of the problem, as the chapters in Part 2 will make clear, lies in the uneven distribution in Peru of facilities, medical personnel, and funds, and part is due to the fact that the public health system, on whom the poor must depend for modern health services, is overburdened by expensive hospital services, undersupplied with medicines, and inefficiently administered. But there is a third aspect to the problem: many middle-class Peruvians, especially those who work for large private sector employers, bypass expensive private sector health care, relying instead on public sector providers, particularly (given the dearth of private sector hospitals) for hospitalization. Thus they add to the financial burden of the already hard-pressed public health care system.

Part of the solution to the medical disenfranchisement of nearly a third of the Peruvian population may lie in increased private health insurance and other prepaid coverage for middle-class Peruvians. This would translate directly into less middle-class utilization of MOH services, and the Ministry could then devote more of its resources to its primary constituency, the medically indigent. Peru has lagged far behind other countries in the LAC region in the development of new forms of health care risk-sharing mechanisms (GHAA 1985), but the last few years have witnessed the emergence of several relatively inexpensive varieties of private health care coverage in which the insurer and provider are the same entity.

The most interesting of the new private prepaid mechanisms are arrangements in which groups of patients (for example, employment-related groups) and/or groups of medical personnel (for example, private medical associations) share in the risk of insuring patients against the costs of injury or illness, sometimes through brokers and sometimes in concert with particular health care facilities, but always for a set, prepaid fee. Referred to as "prepaid, managed health care plans," such insurance mechanisms often combine the financing with the actual delivery of health care, in any of several different ways. This chapter traces the etiology of various private sector health care financing arrangements, describes and compares their current configurations, and assesses their potential for contributing to a solution of Peru's overall health care problems.

Historical Overview

Private health insurance in Peru, a phenomenon almost exclusively restricted to the Lima/Callao area, began to emerge in the late 1970s, as Peru experienced rapid urban growth, economic decline, and deteriorating public health services. With the waning effectiveness and efficiency of public sector health care organizations, dissatisfied employers and unions in the manufacturing and service sectors began to seek alternatives, particularly to the IPSS medical care program. Meanwhile, increasing industrialization was producing a more and more sophisticated labor force, accustomed to receiving company benefits. Employees' welfare funds (*fondos de asistencia y estimulo al trabajador*) were established by law, and some large companies also instituted health funds (HFs). Both of these kinds of financial entities were supported by mandatory contributions from employers and employees (2). Both began to purchase insurance to cover workers' health-related expenditures not covered by IPSS.

Sales of insurance policies through these employment-related welfare and health funds grew rapidly, since (unlike IPSS) they allowed workers to access private providers of their choice promptly and at reasonable cost. (Table 4.1 shows that sales of health policies by insurance companies grew from less than 2 percent of total insurance sales in 1977 to almost 9 percent in 1984.) As inflation in the early 1980s gave way to deep recession in 1982-83, health insurance purchasers—both groups and individual families—were forced to search for less costly and more comprehensive coverage. The market now became very competitive, with several factors contributing to the development of new health care financing and delivery systems. First, the market fragmented as more and more insurance companies entered the field. Second, insurance costs continued to rise as the cost basis used by insurance companies to determine their prices was affected by inflation and by a service tax levied on policy sales (3). And third, the increased cost of premiums put pressure on company health funds either to increase the mandatory contributions of both employers and employees or to seek less costly insurance.

Several health funds bypassed the insurance companies altogether, seeking out, through brokers, administrative and insurance options to traditional commercial health insurance. Two different kinds of broker-managed arrangements (described below) developed, with similarly favorable impacts on reducing the prices of policies and increasing the benefits to welfare and health fund members.

At the same time, health care delivery facilities and providers saw the opportunity to reduce costs and increase earnings by entering into health care coverage contracts directly with company health funds, thus eliminating both brokers and insurance companies. The growth of this type of arrangement was encouraged by two factors. First, health fund administrators had by now gained several years' experience in estimating their beneficiaries' utilization of services and in negotiating with providers. And second, a number of private hospitals and medical groups had been providing health services under contracts with IPSS, insurance companies, or brokers, and their administrative skills, too, had improved. Private hospitals also saw a way to increase their occupancy rates by offering prepayment plans directly to individuals and to groups of people not necessarily related by employment—sometimes with as few as five members.

The recession of 1982-83 thus affected private health care providers completely differently from public sector providers. As public sector health expenditures began to decline, private sector expenditures continued to increase as resources were increasingly transferred from public to private providers in the wake of continuing dissatisfaction with deteriorating MOH and IPSS services. Private health care coverage, in part responsible for this transfer of resources, was an idea whose time had come.

Current Health Insurance Configurations

Private health care coverage involves four essential participants: a financing entity (sometimes referred to, in what follows, as "the plan"), a medical care facility, a medical staff, and a beneficiary, who may be insured as an individual or as a member of a group. In Peru (almost exclusively in the Lima/Callao metropolitan area), relationships between these participants have evolved into three major health insurance configurations: 1) traditional insurance company coverage; 2) coverage through health funds, managed either by employers or for them, by brokers; and 3) prepaid, managed coverage in which the financing and delivery of health care are linked.

Insurance Company Coverage

Eighteen general insurance companies now offer health insurance policies in Lima/Callao. They constitute a fairly homogeneous group in terms of the types of policies offered, benefits, limits of coverage, and relationships with insured persons and providers. Most of their policies represent contracts between insurance companies and groups—usually health funds or other employment-related groups, although they also accept individual enrollments. Premiums are paid directly, by individuals, employers, or employment-related health funds; in the latter case, a part of the premium may be paid by employee contributions.

The benefits packages of insurance company policies are of three types: hospitalization only, hospitalization and medical care, and comprehensive care (including emergency treatment and drugs). Over 75 percent of the policies sold in Lima/Callao are comprehensive. Coverage is usually limited to specific services and always by maximum amounts, and most policies stipulate that enrollees must pay excess charges, coinsurance, deductibles, or copayments of between 10 and 20 percent of the unit costs of services (except for copayments on hospitalization, which are much lower). Costs of treatment beyond the maximum amount covered are usually the responsibility of the individual enrollee, although they are sometimes paid by the enrollee's company welfare or health fund (4).

Generally, this type of insurance does not imply a contractual bond between the insurance company and specific medical personnel or facilities; enrollees are usually free to select from a wide spectrum of providers. Depending on the policy, the insurance company may either pay health care providers directly or may reimburse the enrollees for the costs of services incurred.

Insurance premiums, in principle, are set so as to cover insurance costs plus a reasonable profit, but in practice, they often fail to cover costs, due to inflation. Premiums are generally set at a fixed 4 percent of the total maximum annual face value of the policy. Both premiums and maximum coverage can be adjusted quarterly, depending on utilization, duration of the contract, and the inflation rate. But these adjustments are apt to be unrealistic, as evidenced in recent years by an average cost of claims of over 80 percent of premiums, rather than the targeted 65 percent.

Thus, despite frequent adjustments, insurance companies take a considerable financial gamble on their health insurance policies. In fact, health insurance is now considered to be a poor risk by diversified insurance companies, but they continue to offer it as a "loss leader" with which to attract clients to more profitable kinds of insurance (*e.g.*, fire, shipping, etc.). Companies have tried to increase their profits from health insurance by introducing cost controls, but these have generally consisted only of claims limitations and medical audits of utilization of services. Since the providers of health care do not share the financial risk with the insurance companies, they lack incentives to control costs.

An important achievement of Peruvian insurance companies was the formation of SEGUS (*Seguros Unidos de Salud*), an organization established by seven insurance companies to negotiate common fee schedules with medical personnel and facilities and to coordinate medical audits as a means of controlling utilization of services. These insurance companies now obtain preferential rates—usually 20 percent below regular rates—from both health care facilities and medical groups (see Table 4.2, in which prices are given not in *soles*, the monetary unit in use in Peru prior to 1986, but in *intis*, worth 1000 *soles*, which became the Peruvian monetary unit in 1986). SEGUS also arbitrates disputes between insurance companies and providers, and it is the only institution that collects statistical information about health insurance on a systematic (if limited) basis.

Coverage through Employment-related Health Funds (HFs)

The financing entity in this type of health care coverage is either a large company or a separate entity directly and exclusively related to such an employer. Most Peruvian corporations of over 200 employees now have HFs. (Some of the largest companies plan to develop their own health care facilities, but at present all of them purchase health care services from outside physicians and facilities.) Generally, employees contribute a fixed amount to the HF regardless of the health care expenses they incur. This member contribution only partially covers the cost of the health plan; the company pays the difference.

A health fund can acquire health care coverage for its members in any of three different ways. First, it can obtain a traditional group health policy with an insurance company; the resulting configuration is identical to the insurance company coverage just described. Second, it can obtain a group health plan with an association of physicians or a hospital offering a prepayment arrangement. Finally, it can assume the financial risk itself, purchasing health care services either directly from providers or through an insurance broker who manages the fund's resources and returns any remaining monies to the fund.

The use of a broker as an intermediary has several advantages. The broker negotiates the prices physicians or facilities charge for health services, and may also implement cost control methods such as claims reviews and utilization limits. In addition, brokers sometimes also act as administrators, hired for a fixed fee to manage invoicing, payments, auditing, and utilization control tasks. Finally, they may be financial coinsurers, a variant on HF coverage discussed below under "Broker-managed Health Funds."

Most HFs arrange for their members to receive health care at one or more private hospitals or clinics, provided by the staffs of these facilities' associated medical groups. In order to obtain preferred rates, HFs generally award contracts to medical groups and facilities through a bidding process, with rates typically fixed for a period of two to five years. A patient's choice of physicians and facilities is thus limited, sometimes to the extent that he or she can obtain health care from only one clinic or hospital and its associated medical group. Members are treated according to a specific schedule of benefits, and the HF is billed accordingly. The range of health services covered is usually quite comprehensive, although there is wide variation with regard to dental care and the provision of drugs.

Since in this configuration there is no inherent reason why users and providers should restrict their utilization or provision of services (similar to the insurance company problem), most HFs have established financial deterrents to discourage overutilization. A few specify deductibles, but most require copayments in the form of flat fees-per-service. These are generally lower than those required under standard insurance company policies.

A variant of health fund coverage is the broker-managed health fund, similar to the arrangement described immediately above except that the HF hires a broker who has absolute control over the fund. If the fund's resources exceed the expenses incurred by its enrollees, the broker keeps the difference as his profit. If, however, the expenses incurred by the users exceed the fund's resources, the HF, rather than the broker, pays the difference. The broker thus assumes no risk; it is the HF that bears the risk. This configuration introduces an important new element into the relationship among the four agents involved in health insurance: incentives to control costs. Since his profits depend on effective control of services utilization, the broker is powerfully motivated to control costs by negotiating predetermined fees and supervising the utilization of services.

Prepaid Financing/Delivery Plans

These insurance arrangements differ from the insurance company and HF configurations in that they directly link insurers with the facilities at which health care is provided, and sometimes with medical personnel as well. Thus the insurance plan is closely associated with a private hospital or clinic, and in some cases a specific medical group (5). The financing agent (the private facility or an entity directly associated with it) offers health coverage to individuals or employment-related groups. The enrollees, whether individuals, families, or groups, receive coverage for a predetermined premium regardless of the amount of consumption of health care services. The prices of premiums vary from plan to plan, but are usually influenced by the desire of prepaid financing/delivery plans' administrators to maintain a competitive edge in the marketplace (6).

In Lima/Callao, the four currently-existing plans that conform to the prepaid financing/delivery configuration take one of three forms, differing according to who bears the risk: the medical facility alone, the facility and a group of medical personnel, or the facility and a medical group plus a nominally separate financing entity.

In *Type A*, represented by Clinicas San Borja and San Felipe, the financing entity is the clinic, which is separate from the staff of medical personnel who supply the actual health care. Enrollees pay the clinic a fixed monthly premium regardless of their consumption of services, thereby transferring the financial risk of possible illness to the clinic. The clinic pays its associated physicians individually, on a fee-for-service basis, for providing enrollees with the services included in the benefits schedule. Upon consumption of services, the enrollees pay a small copayment, stipulated in the contract. Since the clinic receives no formal payment for the services it provides to the enrollees, its profits or losses depend on two factors: ambulatory care service utilization (generally beyond the clinic's control), and hospitalization expenses (which the clinic may partially control through an efficient use of resources). Overutilization and overproduction of services are encouraged by low copayments, by the method used to pay physicians, and by the fact that the system does not incorporate the actual providers of care.

In *Type B*, represented by Clinica Anglo-Americana, the financing entity is again a clinic, again separate from the physicians who provide health care to the enrollees. The physicians, however, belong to a formal association, which is paid a fixed amount per enrollee per month regardless of the enrollees' consumption of services. The physicians' association, in turn, pays its members for the services provided by each. Payment is made according to a point system, in which excessive utilization of services reduces the monetary value of each service. As in Type A, the clinic does not receive payment for hospitalization services provided to the enrollees; its profit or loss depends on the ratio of subscription income to the hospitalization expenses of the insured, which the clinic may partially control through an efficient use of its resources. Thus the financial risk is assumed jointly by the clinic and the physicians, with the clinic's risk somewhat greater since its influence over physicians is more limited than the influence they may exert over the clinic through their medical decisions. (For example, doctors—not clinics—decide on hospitalization and length of stay.) Since neither the clinic nor the physicians gain from it, overutilization of services is discouraged.

In *Type C*, represented by Clinica Maison de Sante, the financing entity is officially separate from both the clinic and the doctors' association, but these three separate entities are actually interrelated so as to form a single provider organization. The plan pays both the facility and the medical group (which in both cases is closely associated with the facility) on a negotiated fee-for-service basis, regardless of utilization and/or actual cost. Theoretically, the plan assumes all risks; its profit and losses are directly related to the health care and hospitalization expenses incurred by the enrollees. In practice, however, the risk is shared by the three organizations, since they all operate as one entity. In spite of the fact that payments are made on a fee-for-service basis, the *de facto* incorporation of the clinic and physicians into the plan is a disincentive to the overproduction of services.

There are a number of similarities among prepaid financing/delivery plans and both traditional health insurance and HF coverage. Most prepaid financing/delivery plans set limitations on coverage by means of maximum expenditures/enrollee/year as well as maximum amounts for particular services (7). Like health insurance policies, most prepaid financing/delivery plans accept individual enrollment, although groups of at least three members are typical. Most have established deterrents to preclude overutilization—"hesitation fees" or copayments required of enrollees at the time of consumption of services (8). The benefits, like those offered by the HFs, are comprehensive, and include emergency care and drugs prescribed during hospitalization. Dental care and drugs for ambulatory patients are not included.

Of the various configurations, prepaid financing/delivery plans place the greatest limitations on the enrollee's choice of providers (9); the choice is limited to the physicians who are members of the medical group and/or facility associated with or sponsoring the plan, a limitation that may be offset by higher quality or greater continuity of care. Since choice of provider is a feature that beneficiaries value highly, proposals have been made to establish prepaid financing/delivery plans with multiple providers of both ambulatory and hospital care, but at present all four such plans in Lima are limited to one sponsoring facility and one medical group.

Other Plans

As of 1986, several other managed, prepaid health coverage plans were being offered in the Lima/Callao area, but these lacked the direct insurer/provider linkage characterizing the four prepaid financing/delivery plans just described. One, sponsored by a medical center (10), was offering extensive ambulatory care at the center and hospitalization benefits through contracts with private hospitals. Other plans offered health services similar to those available through cooperatives; one (11) offered a 20-30 percent fee discount to members of its "hospital club," while several guilds and specialized associations (12) also offered a limited range of discounted health services with membership. Finally, a local financial institution had recently begun to offer a plan under which individuals with accounts at the institution (similar to a savings and loan) could opt to have part of the interest earned on their deposits applied toward the cost of a health insurance policy premium. The cost and benefits of this premium were similar to conventional insurance policies. Apparently, the financial institution assumed all risks.

Comparative Analysis of Prepayment Alternatives

In order to assess the future of health care insurance and prepayment alternatives, it is necessary first to compare the four most salient features of the currently-existing mechanisms: their risk-sharing arrangements, the benefits they offer for premiums charged, cost control incentives under each configuration, and the present market share of each configuration.

Assumption of Risk

In all health care prepayment mechanisms, individuals pass their risk of incurring medical costs to an institution, which pools subscribers' risks as well as their premium payments. With traditional health insurance, the enrollee pays a fixed amount to the insurance company, thus transferring the financial risk of a possible illness to the company—to the extent specified in the policy. Theoretically, this configuration is the least risky to the insurer, since the amount of risk the insurer is obliged to take in the event of an enrollee's illness or injury is limited under the terms of every policy. Costs in excess of the stipulated amount are invariably borne by the enrollee. In reality, however, the insurance company's risk may be considerable, particularly in times of rapidly-rising inflation, since the premiums paid by enrollees may be insufficient to cover the costs of claims.

Under the self-administered health fund configuration, members transfer some or all of the financial risk of possible illness to the fund. Some HFs have set a maximum amount of coverage per beneficiary per period of time, while others provide unlimited coverage. HFs generally assume a larger proportion of financial risk than insurance companies do, and in those cases in which the extent of coverage is unlimited, HFs bear the most risk of all the insurance alternatives. Some charge employees for costs in excess of stipulated maximum coverage, but the most common arrangement is for the fund to pay excess costs itself or to recover them from employees in monthly installments.

When a health fund is managed by a broker, it also shares the risk of insuring employees with the broker. The broker's risk is minimal, however, for he is responsible for paying providers for their services only up to the actual amount with which the HF has entrusted him. If the cost of claims surpasses this amount, the broker seeks the difference from the fund (which must in turn get it from the beneficiaries). The broker's only real risk, therefore, is that he might not make a profit over and above the fixed fee he charges the HF for his services.

Under the prepaid financing/delivery configuration, risk is apportioned differently under the three different models. In the Type A organization, in which the plan and health care facility are a single entity with which the medical personnel are not formally associated, the risk is assumed by the facility/plan, within limits described in the policy. The physicians, who are paid on a fee-for service basis, take no risk. Type B involves a facility/plan and physicians who, while not associated with the facility, are formally incorporated into a medical group which receives a fixed payment per enrollee from the plan. The medical group is paid on a *per capita* basis, regardless of the number and value of services rendered to enrollees. If the cost of services provided to beneficiaries is greater than the amount raised in premiums, the resulting loss cannot be passed to another organization or back to the consumer. The risk is thus shared by the facility sponsoring the plan and the medical group, although the facility bears a somewhat larger share since it is legally responsible for the plan and since its performance can be affected by the decisions of its physicians concerning who will be hospitalized, for what, and for how long. Type C involves a facility, a medical group, and a separate financing entity that in effect form a single organization. The plan pays both the facility and the medical group on a fee-for-service basis. Although on paper the financial risk is assumed solely by the plan, in reality—since the three institutions form a single organization—gains and losses are shared.

Benefits and Premiums

In metropolitan Lima/Callao, the insurance and prepaid health care market has many variations in premium prices and benefits coverage, despite the recent efforts of several insurance companies, through SEGUS, to standardize policies. This diversity can be viewed as evidence of competition through product differentiation, although it may also be a product of inadequate information.

In Table 4.3, premiums and extent of coverage are compared among traditional health insurance, brokered HF coverage, non-brokered HF coverage, and prepaid financing/delivery plans. Monthly premiums range from 27 *intis*, in a low-option health insurance policy, to a high-option plan offered by a broker at 450 *intis*. The differences in benefits, of course, are likely to be considerable, although there is no systematic information on the basis of which one might compare benefits and costs among plans.

In 1986, the prepaid financing/delivery plans in Lima/Callao were serving very different populations. The most expensive and prestigious (13) served a small group of upper-income clients with a limited schedule of benefits. Two others (14) together provided services to the largest group of users, approximately 25,000 middle-income enrollees, at a high-premium, limited-benefits rate. One (15), with 14,000 enrollees, predominantly served a lower-income population.

With one exception (16), all the prepaid financing/ delivery policies specify coverage limitations. Most health fund and prepaid financing/delivery plans also require "hesitation payments" or copayments for hospitalization, ambulatory care, diagnostic tests, and ambulance services. Employer health plans typically exclude from coverage congenital conditions, psychiatric services, regular physical exams, plastic surgery for esthetic reasons, orthopedic prostheses, dental care, ophthalmological services, pregnancy and prenatal care, drug addiction, injury due to civil disturbances, suicide attempts, injuries due to treatment performed by non-physicians, blood products, and nursing care. In all plans, enrollment of new members is generally limited to those 65 and under (17). Frequently, a physical exam is a prerequisite to enrollment, and can be used to deny admittance to a plan. Most policies become effective within 30 days of enrollment (18).

Cost Control Incentives

As with other aspects of the various kinds of health care coverage, there is wide variety in cost control incentives among the various plans.

Under insurance company policies, consumers—whose costs for using private medical care are substantially lowered by insurance—are thus encouraged to consume more services; deterrents (copayments and deductibles) and a limit to the amount of coverage per type of service help to curb overutilization. Physicians, paid on a fee-for-service basis, do not have strong incentives to control abuse of the system, since the more services they deliver and the more expensive those services are, the higher their incomes. The insurance company payment method may thus encourage unnecessary utilization, which should ultimately raise costs. In Lima's highly competitive insurance market, however, insurance companies find it difficult to pass increased costs on to consumers, and are thus forced to consider stronger cost-control measures. Several Peruvian companies have taken steps in this direction, including cooperative action through SEGUS. In addition, a recent trend toward providing more ambulatory care through group practices, as an alternative to hospitalization, can be viewed as a cost-control measure.

Since health funds, whether self-run or broker-managed, charge enrollees a set amount and typically pay medical personnel on a fee-for-service basis, the structure of incentives is similar to that described for insurance companies: neither enrollees nor providers have strong reasons to limit their use of the system, although the process of bidding for service contracts with particular hospitals or clinics does lower the cost of these establishments' services. Cost-control measures undertaken by self-run HFs include reviews of the appropriateness of claims, utilization reviews, the identification of heavy users, and medical audits, but without any sharing of financial risk with providers, HFs' control over the costs of service is limited (19).

For prepaid financing/delivery plans, three different risk-bearing entities have been identified:

In Type A, the plan and facility are incorporated into a single institution, but the physicians have individual contractual arrangements with the plan and are paid on a fee-for-service basis. The facility receives no per-patient payment, since it is part of the same organization as the plan. Several elements may contribute to overutilization: the method of remuneration of physicians, the absence of organized procedures typical of a managed care setting, and very low copayments.

In Type B, which involves a plan and hospital as parts of the same institution but physicians who are formally incorporated into a medical group and paid on a *per capita* basis, regardless of the number and value of services they provide to enrollees, there are deterrents to the overutilization of medical services. Each physician in the medical group is paid for services on a sliding scale. In addition, a strong peer review system exists among the physicians, which helps to insure that only needed services are provided.

In Type C, the plan, facility, and physicians' association are three separate entities. In theory, neither the hospital nor the medical group has incentives to control utilization and costs. Nevertheless, since the three entities are interrelated, the actual risk is shared by all, which restrains them from overproducing services.

Present Market Shares

The number of people covered by private sector insurance and prepayment arrangements in the Lima/Callao area is difficult to estimate due to a scarcity of information. There are few data on either the number of policies sold or the number of people protected; even SEGUS has serious difficulties in obtaining data from the very companies that created it. No regulation mandates that brokers, health funds, or the administrators of prepaid financing/delivery plans report either the volume of their sales or number of persons covered to any agency.

In order to produce a market share estimate, we first used the total 1985 sales of health insurance by insurance companies and the prevailing price of an average individual policy to estimate the number of people covered by insurance companies, based on the largest-selling policy of the insurance company with the most sales (20). The total volume of sales of health insurance policies by all insurance companies for 1985 was estimated at 101.64 million *intis* (21), and the number of insurance company policies sold in 1985 was (conservatively) estimated to be about 47,700. Since the average policy covered 4.5 people, the number of persons who could have been covered by insurance companies in 1985 was around 215,000. Second, managers who were interviewed suggested that health funds represent a similar number of persons, adding another 215,000 to the size of the privately-insured population. Finally, it was estimated, based on interviews with administrators of the provider-managed plans, that these four plans together enroll about 40,000 individuals.

The 1985 total for all types of insurance was thus about 470,000 people, of whom 45 percent were covered by insurance companies, 45 percent by health funds, and 10 percent by prepaid financing/delivery plans. These figures are in accordance with the estimates of interviewees from the health insurance field in Lima/Callao, who all produced figures in the range of 400,000-600,000 enrollees. If these figures are correct (and we believe they are), the total coverage of households by some form of private health insurance or prepaid plans in Peru is only 4 percent.

Conclusions

At present, the Peruvian private health insurance market is very small, and is dominated by insurance companies and self-financed company health funds. Recently, however, several kinds of prepaid, managed health care plans, in which the financing of health care is combined with its actual delivery, have developed in Lima. These plans are associated with particular health care facilities, and all (like health maintenance organizations in the United States) charge prepaid fees. If more such plans were to develop in Peru, and if they were to charge lower premium prices, the market for them would expand. Indeed, a continuation of the recent trend toward more private coverage under all of these risk-sharing mechanisms appears likely. This should help to alleviate the problem of the heavy use by middle-class Peruvians of public sector providers, particularly for hospitalization, and would thus help to relieve the financial burden of the hard-pressed public health care system.

But two *caveats* are in order. First, employees of the largest companies in Peru—those that pay relatively high salaries and have the strongest management and union leadership—already have health care coverage, either through private health insurance or company-managed health funds. Significant growth in private sector coverage, therefore, will also require that more, and more efficient, prepaid financing/delivery plans, such as the four provider-managed plans analyzed in this chapter, emerge to help create and satisfy the potential demand of families and small special-interest groups for low-cost, prepaid health care coverage. And second, the private sector, if it is to offer coverage under insurance or prepayment arrangements, will have to provide more hospital services than it currently controls. This does not necessarily mean that more hospitals will have to be built; instead, the public sector could turn over some of its hospital facilities to private sector management.

Footnotes

1. This chapter is based on HCF/LAC 1987, which in turn drew upon statistical data available from previous research efforts and descriptive reports (HSA-Peru 1986).

2. Most health funds now receive equal contributions from employers and employees.

3. To remain financially viable, insurance companies cannot pay costs for claims in excess of 65 percent of total premium income. Another 30 percent is

set aside for administrative costs and brokers' commissions, and there is a 5 percent profit. The insurance companies must also charge an 11 percent sales tax, passed on to the consumer.

4. It is estimated that over 60 percent of all insured patients requiring hospitalization incur hospital costs greater than the maximum amount covered under their policies.

5. As of 1986, this arrangement was offered by only four health care facilities in Lima: Clinica San Borja, Clinica San Felipe, Clinica Anglo-Americana, and the Club de Salud at the Clinica Maison de Sante, jointly with the clinic's Associacion de Medicos Miguel Aljovin. Of the three different types of prepaid financing/delivery plans to be described in this chapter, San Borja and San Felipe are representative of the first, Anglo-Americana of the second, and Maison de Sante of the third.

6. One plan (Maison de Sante), however, has significantly lower prices, due to its special philanthropic orientation.

7. Only one currently-existing plan assumes all risk and offers unlimited coverage.

8. The plan of the Maison de Sante's Club de la Salud has no deterrent fees, since in the opinion of its management this would defeat the purpose of the arrangement: to remove financial barriers to high quality care.

9. Freedom of choice is strongly defended by the medical profession. Apparently, prepayment plans are acceptable to the profession because a choice is made among physicians at the time one joins a plan.

10. Los Pinos.

11. The Clinica Ricardo Palma.

12. For example, Ambulancia San Cristobal.

13. Clinica Anglo-Americana.

14. San Borja and San Felipe.

15. The Maison de Sante.

16. Again, the Maison de Sante.

17. Except for the Maison de Sante, which has no age limit but does charge a higher premium rate for the elderly.

18. The Maison de Sante permits certain benefits immediately upon enrollment, and gradually increases coverage to 100 percent over a period of four months.

19. Only one instance was found in which a health fund had transferred risk to providers: a fund at Hierro Peru, under a contract with the Clinica Anglo-Americana. In this case, the HF pays the Clinica (which operates a prepayment plan of its own) a flat amount/beneficiary/month, independent of the total cost of services used.

20. El Pacifico.

21. This figure reflects sales of health insurance in the entire country; there is no data available specifically for Lima/Callao. However, since almost all health insurance policies were sold in the metropolitan area, it is appropriate to assume that the value for the country is applicable to the metropolitan area.

TABLE 4.1

Private Health Insurance Sales, 1977 - 84
(in thousands of constant 1980 soles)

	1977	1978	1979	1980	1981	1982	1983	1984
All Policies								
Gross Insurance Sales	63,809	55,251	54,699	60,961	62,803	62,100	59,100	60,613
Reinsurance Costs	39,409	33,517	33,673	36,757	37,069	31,693	32,574	31,938
Net Sales	24,399	21,734	21,026	24,204	25,734	30,407	26,526	28,676
Health Policies								
Gross Insurance Sales	1,117	1,206	1,811	2,430	3,231	3,929	3,262	3,511
Reinsurance Costs	89	45	0	0	0	22	22	27
Net Sales	1,028	1,161	1,811	2,430	3,231	3,907	3,240	3,484
Health policies as % of total	1.86	2.45	3.61	4.31	5.53	6.79	6.05	8.80

Source: Government of Peru 1977-84.

TABLE 4.2

Private Hospital: Example of Fee Schedules for Different Users
(prices in intis as of July 1986)

		Rates	
		Preferred (insurance rate)	Regular
Hospital room:			
New building:	Private, with phone	250.00	275.00
	Private, without phone	220.00	240.00
Old building:	Private, without phone	200.00	220.00
	Semi-private (shared bath)	160.00	180.00
	Wards (4 or 6 beds)	130.00	150.00
Intensive care	(per 24 hours)	540.00	600.00
Operating room:			
Initial half hour		250.00	280.00
Second half hour		230.00	250.00
Each additional half hour		120.00	140.00
Physician:	Medical assistant		
Surgery:	less than half hour	120.00	200.00
Surgery:	upto one hour	130.00	250.00
Surgery:	over one hour	150.00	300.00
Surgical procedures:			
Tonsilectomy -	operating room	250.00	300.00
	Medical assistant	120.00	150.00

Source: A private hospital with lower than average rates.

TABLE 4.3

Price of Premium and Maximum Coverage for Selected Health Insurance Mechanisms—Lima, Peru, 1986

(Prices in intis as of July 1986)

	Premium Cost of Policyholder	Premium Cost of Policyholder + 1 dependent	Premium Cost of Policyholder + 2 dependents	Maximum Coverage	Ratio (%)*
HEALTH INSURANCE COMPANIES					
ItalSeguros	51	130	171	10,000	1.7
Segusfa	59	92	131	7,800	1.6
Financiera Progreso	95	275	350	30,000	1.2
El Pacifico (1)	27	75	122	10,000	1.2
BROKER'S POLICIES					
Broker (A)	195	326	387	30,000	1.3
Broker (B)	425	682	772	80,000	1.0
Broker (C)	450	734	832	100,000	0.8
HEALTH FUND					
Banco de la Nacion	110	220	330	8,700	3.8
PREPAID FINANCING/DELIVERY PLANS					
Anglo - Americana	95	190	285	9,500	3.0
Maison Sante (A)	48	83	110	Unlimited	N/A
Maison Sante (B)	82	136	180	Unlimited	N/A
San Borja (A)	98	146	204	10,400	2.0
San Borja (B)	112	224	336	15,400	2.2

Source: Company brochures, 1986.

Note: (1) Data for May 1985
(2) The amount contributed as "premium" by the beneficiaries of the Health Fund is only 20% of the total premium cost. Thus, the total cost per beneficiary per per month is used in the table.

* Ratio of policyholder and 2 dependents to maximum coverage.

PART TWO

Resources Allocation and Policy Implications

5

Distribution of Health Care Facilities

Ethel R. Carrillo

Over the past five years, Peru's health policies have been directed toward two important goals: a reorientation of the health sector toward primary health care (PHC), which incorporates preventive as well as curative care, and improvements in the distribution of health care facilities throughout the country. An analysis of the types, distribution, accessibility, and potential capacity of Peru's health care facilities, however, shows that hospitals, and hence hospital beds, are heavily concentrated in the major urban areas, and that primary health care facilities—although more equitably distributed—are insufficient in number and poorly maintained.

This chapter provides a population-based analysis of the distribution and potential capacity of different types health care facilities in Peru. First, Peru's geographical areas, political divisions, and population distribution and density and described, and related to the structure of the health care delivery system as of 1985. The chapter then analyzes the availability of and potential need for hospital beds, assessing coverage at the departmental, regional, and hospital-area levels. The present availability of health care facilities at the departmental level is compared with the situation that existed in 1975, so that significant changes over a ten-year period can be identified. After the results of a 1985 survey on the physical status of facilities, utility systems, and equipment in the health regions of Cajamarca and Cuzco are presented, the chapter ends with an assessment of the possibilities for improving access to health care for the less favored segments of Peru's population.

The analysis is based on a selection of data available in their entirety in HSA-Peru 1986e. The selected data, as well as the specific indicators used in the study, are given at the regional and hospital area levels, as well as by department (1). It is important to point out that the data on the population density of hospital areas were developed specifically for this study, based on demographic and geographic information by district (the smallest political division in Peru) supplied by the National Institute of Statistics (INE) and the National Planning Institute (INP). The individual sections of the chapter take as their units of analysis either departments or health regions and hospital areas.

Geopolitical and Health Administrative Divisions

From a health services perspective, the major ecological zones of Peru—the coast, *sierra* (mountains), and jungle—are vastly different from one another, both in terms of population density and living standards. The coast, in general, is the most densely populated as well as the most urbanized zone, and enjoys the highest standards of living and life expectancies (see Chapter 2). Living conditions in the (primarily rural) *sierra* and jungle are, on the whole, poorer, and population density is much lower (Table 5.1).

Politically, Peru is divided into 25 principal units: 24 departments and one constitutional province (Callao, which in Table 5.1 has been incorporated into the department of Lima). These vary widely in terms of geographic area, population numbers, and population density (Table 5.1).

From 1982 to 1985, the Ministry of Health (MOH) divided the country into "health regions" that were not contiguous with departmental boundaries. These health regions were further divided into "hospital areas." It was hoped that this reorganization of health services would help to bring about the decentralization of what had long been an intensely centralized health care delivery system, and would thus assure greater equity of access to health care across the entire Peruvian population. The system proved ineffective, however, and in 1985 was abandoned in favor of a return to department-level administration of health services, but with a stronger emphasis on community participation at the local level (see Chapter 3).

As the theoretical framework for the analysis and results presented in this chapter, we used a pyramidal health care referral scheme in which small local facilities provide referrals to larger regional facilities, which in turn refer patients to major hospitals where specialized treatment is available. To use the World Health Organization (WHO) terminology (Hogart 1978), there are three basic types of facilities: hospitals, health centers, and health posts. Among hospitals there are significant differences depending on their regional or local orientation and their degree of specialization. In order for the referral system to function properly, each section of the country (department or health region) must have a complementary array of facilities consisting of a relatively large number of health posts, somewhat fewer health centers, and proportionately even fewer hospitals.

Ideally, a potential patient first seeks help at a local health post or health center within his hospital area (2). Health posts are located mainly in disadvantaged urban, suburban, and rural areas, where they provide preventive medical care, health education, and emergency treatment; health centers, functionally related to local or regional hospitals, act as satellites, providing medical consultations, minor surgery, odontological care, vaccinations, and educational programs. Some health centers have beds for emergency hospitalization; some do not.

If the patient's medical condition justifies it, s/he is referred from the health post or health center to an intermediate-sized facility—a local or regional hospital. These are located in the largest city of each of the hospital areas and regions, respectively, and provide general medical, surgical, gynecological/ obstetrical, and pediatric care. In theory, regional hospitals should also have additional specialized departments, such as neurosurgery, plastic surgery, and radiotherapy, with enough capacity to serve the entire region.

Finally, if adequate treatment is not possible at the regional level, the patient is referred to a major urban hospital in which there is a department specializing in the treatment of his or her specific health care needs.

Health Care Facilities and Population Distribution

The division of Peruvian health sector resources into public and private subsectors—and the further division of resources, within the public subsector, among MOH, IPSS, the uniformed forces, and other (*e.g.*, parastatal) health services—was outlined in Chapter 1. Each of these institutional categories is responsible for the operation of health care facilities of the three different kinds just described. In 1985, the facilities available, by category, were as follows:

	Sector		MOH		IPSS		Uniformed Forces and Other Public		Private	
	No.	%	No.	%	No.	%	No.	%	No.	%
HB	29,984	100	16,183	54	4,730	16	3,687	12	5,384	18
HC	785	100	612	78	34	4	101	13	38	5
HP	1,925	100	1,712	89	33	2	99	5	81	4

Note: HB = hospital beds; HC = health centers; HP = health posts Source: Table 5.2

The combined public sector shares of hospital beds (82 percent), health centers (95 percent), and health posts (90 percent) illustrate the predominance of the public sector in the delivery of health care, although there is virtually no coordination in the planning or operation of the major institutional categories of public health services.

The geographical and departmental distribution of the Peruvian population, and its density, are shown in Table 5.1. Note the intense concentration of Peruvians in the coastal departments (particularly in Lima/Callao) and their sparse distribution in other departments. In the sprawling Lima/Callao metropolitan area, there are approximately 6 million Peruvians, with a density of 184 people per square kilometer. In sharp contrast are the population densities of rural departments in the jungle zone, particularly Madre de Dios, Loreto, and Ucayali (less than two inhabitants per square kilometer).

Table 5.2 shows the number (by department) and institutional affiliation of all health care facilities in Peru (see ANSSA-Peru 1986f, Anexo 2). Several points are of particular interest here. First, the overall numbers of health posts (1,925), health centers (785), and hospitals (338) suggest that the Peruvian health services system is quite well-balanced. But a closer look at the table shows that this balance breaks down at the departmental level. Moquegua, for instance, with a population density of 7.41 persons per km^2 (Table 5.1), has 376 hospital beds, while Cajamarca, with a much higher density of 33.14, has only 246 beds. The ratio of population to hospital beds in most of the country's departments is inversely related to the distribution of population (see Table 5.3); in fact, 19 of Peru's 24 departments have higher population-to-bed ratios than the national average. This disproportionate distribution is particularly strong in Cajamarca and the departments in the southern *sierra*.

Second, the concentration of hospitals (38 percent of Peru's total)—and especially of hospital beds (55 percent)—in the Lima/Callao area is disproportionate to the relative size of this area's population (31 percent of the country's total). This concentration of hospitals includes not only MOH and IPSS institutions but also uniformed forces and private facilities, all of which concentrate over 50 percent of their hospital beds in Lima/Callao.

And third, there is considerable overlap in the subsectorial provision of facilities. With the exception of the MOH, all other institutions have most of their hospitals located in the major coastal departments: Lima/Callao, Arequipa, La Libertad, Lambayeque, and Piura, while departments like Amazonas, Madre de Dios, and Tumbes each have only one relatively small hospital.

Health centers are more evenly distributed in relation to population distribution than hospitals, but they still show substantial variation among departments (Table 5.3). There are six departments whose population percentages are much larger than their share of health centers: Apurimac, Ayacucho, Cajamarca, Cuzco, Huanuco, and Puno. All are typically disadvantaged highland areas.

Finally, it can be seen from Table 5.3 that the geographical location of health posts is also considerably more equitable, in relation to population distribution, than that of hospital beds. Since health posts, however, depend on health centers and hospitals for referral services, supplies, and supervision within the pyramidal structure of a health services system, the disequilibrium in the availability of the respective facilities suggests that health posts, though adequate in number, may not function very effectively in regions where they are not within ready access to higher levels of care.

Table 5.4 shows the percentages of total health facilities operated by the MOH. It is obvious that the MOH is the most important of Peru's health care delivery institutions, managing 35 percent of all the sector's hospitals and 54 percent of all hospital beds, as well as 78 percent and 89 percent, respectively, of health centers and posts. Table 5.4 also demonstrates that the Ministry's hospital infrastructure is highly concentrated in Lima/Callao (49 percent of all beds), but that the distribution of MOH health centers and posts better corresponds to the population distribution.

Physical Infrastructure and Distribution Network

We have noted that, for the sector as a whole, the proportions of hospitals, health centers and health posts in Peru are consistent with a pyramidal referral structure toward which the country's health policy has been directed for the past five to ten years. Moreover, the total number of hospital beds in Peru—almost 30,000—appears adequate for a population of close to 20 million people (in 1985). However, the distributions of the different types of health care facilities by health regions and hospital areas is highly unbalanced. Broadly speaking, facilities tend to be concentrated in the health regions serving Lima/Callao and other cities of the urbanized coastal departments, while most rural health regions are underserved.

The 17 health regions of Peru are identified in Table 5.5, showing all health sector facilities located in each region and hospital area. Ideally, each region should contain coordinated services, by levels. However, because there is little or no relationship between the administrative denomination of hospitals and their actual characteristics (there are "regional" hospitals, for instance, in a great variety of sizes), we have classified Peruvian hospitals by size, following MOH standards (MOH 1982), as follows:

Type 1: up to 50 beds
Type 2: 51 to 150 beds
Type 3: 151 to 300 beds
Type 4: 301 or more beds

An analysis of the distribution of hospitals by type shows that in 12 of the 17 health regions there are no Type 4 hospitals (Table 5.5). These very large hospitals are found only in the coastal cities, and are heavily concentrated in Lima/Callao. The capital area has 16 of the country's 19 Type 4 hospitals, each with an average of 657 beds. There are no Type 3 (much less Type 4) hospitals in three health regions—Cajamarca, Ayacucho, and Moyabamba. In all hospital areas, however, there is at least one hospital of Type 1 or Type 2. Yet the heaviest concentration of these smaller hospitals (like large ones) is also in the metropolitan Lima/Callao area, which has 25 percent of all Type 1 hospitals. In contrast, 19 of 62 hospital areas have only one hospital of any type (see Table 5.5).

While there is some evidence of a structured network of different types of hospitals for the country as a whole (in that there are fewer large hospitals relative to smaller ones), the proportion of small to large hospitals differs greatly among regions. For example, the ratio of Type 1 to Type 2 hospitals is in some cases equal or close to one, whereas in other areas it is as high as five Type 1 to Type 2 facilities. This suggests that no standard criteria were used in building hospitals in all health regions.

The MOH operates at least one hospital in all hospital areas. However, the ratio of Type 1 to Type 2 MOH hospitals is less consistent than for the entire health sector, since in some cases it is less than one: *e.g.*, there are more large hospitals than small ones under the Ministry's aegis. These observations lead to the conclusion that while a fairly consistent network of hospital facilities exists for the Peruvian health sector as a whole, this is not true for each major institution—and especially not for the MOH, which has the largest responsibility in terms of population coverage: close to 60 percent (see Chapter 1).

The number of health centers for the sector as a whole, moreover, is disproportionately large in most of "central" hospital areas—those considered as regional headquarters (Table 5.5). For example, in Region 4, the Trujillo hospital area has 32 of the region's 36 health centers. The analysis is, however, more meaningful if these figures are related to demographic density.

The health center per unit of population density indicator (HC/pop. density) confirms the scarcity of health centers in some hospital areas. Three-fourths of all hospital areas have relatively few health centers for their highly concentrated populations (see HSA-Peru 1986e:7). Considering their high population densities, these areas may require more health centers, relative to areas with lower population densities (subject, of course, to other considerations). It is interesting to note that HC/pop. density ratios for metropolitan Lima (shown as "Rimac" in Table 5.5, which includes five hospital areas) and Callao are the lowest in the country. This suggests that the population of these adjacent areas has a limited choice of health facilities: many people must seek medical care at hospitals, since the number of health centers available is relatively low because of the high population density. On the other hand, it is important to note that the hospital areas located in the jungle have the highest HC/pop. density ratios (see Iquitos and Madre de Dios, Table 5.5), in part because the population is widely dispersed in that geographic zone. In a comparison at the regional level, five regions were found to have relatively low HC/population density ratios: Cajamarca, Trujillo, Lima, Ayacucho, and Callao.

If instead of applying to the entire health sector the analysis were limited to the MOH, it would lead to roughly the same conclusions. Although the ratios are lower, the regions and areas in greatest need of more facilities are the same (see HSA-Peru 1986e).

For all health posts (89 percent of which are administered by the MOH), a different distribution pattern exists. The health posts to health center (HP/HC) ratio (see Table 5.5) shows that the central hospital areas are not always the most favored. This is as it should be, since health posts have been constructed mainly in the disadvantaged periurban and outlying rural areas. The data also show that the hospital areas of Lima and Callao have the lowest HP/HC indices; for example, Lima (see Rimac in Table 5.5) has a 0.24 ratio, vs. a 2.45 national average). This further supports our earlier observation that residents of this metropolitan area are heavily dependent upon hospital-based services.

When the ratio of health posts per unit of population density (HP/pop. density) (see Table 5.5) is taken into consideration, the situation is somewhat different. Using this ratio demonstrates that most central hospital areas have higher HP/pop. density ratios than do the primarily rural hospital areas, in contrast to what the HP/HC ratio showed. This is true in the central hospital areas of Piura, Cajamarca, Huaraz, Puno, San Martin, and Iquitos. Hospital areas with the worst situations (*i.e.*, with the lowest HP/population density ratios) are Chota, Pacasmayo, Pomabamba, Lima, Tarma, Junin, and Callao. Clearly, Chota, Rimac (Lima), and Callao are in need not only of more health centers but also of more health posts, especially if the Ministry's objective is to reduce the burden placed by these deficits on overloaded hospital outpatient services.

Availability of and Potential Need for Hospital Beds

The conclusion that too many large hospitals have been built, and that their services exceed actual need for inpatient care, would in itself be misleading. It would be correct only if the Peruvian population had ready access to properly-located and equipped smaller hospitals, health centers, and posts.

Large urban hospitals will remain crowded as long as there is no network of facilities to support a referral system in the major population centers, particularly Lima/Callao. Conversely, disadvantaged health regions and hospital areas suffer from a deficit of both PHC facilities (HCs and HPs) and hospitals at the next higher level of a balanced referral system. The systematic analysis of currently-available hospitals is important because of their enormous concentration in a few hospital areas, and because of the uncoordinated actions of the major public sector providers, all of which emphasize tertiary-level instead of primary health care. The following analysis focuses on the number of hospital bed-days available in the health sector as a whole, and specifically in MOH facilities and the potential need of the Peruvian population for those hospital beds (3).

The results, shown in Table 5.6, indicate that, at the sectorial level, there are five health regions with an excess supply of hospital beds: Lima, Callao, Ica, Arequipa, and Tacna. At the other extreme are the regions of Cajamarca, Cuzco, Puno, and Piura, where the need for beds greatly exceeds their supply. As Table 5.6 shows, in some of the regions where there is excess demand the shortage of beds is minimal, and does not justify the construction of new large hospitals.

At the hospital area level, we find more geographically precise illustrations of the situation and its complexities. For example, the Ica and Arequipa health regions both show an excess supply of beds, but the most depressed hospital areas within these regions (Lucanas and Castilla, respectively) have a shortage.

Several Latin American countries have achieved an average length of hospital stay (ALOS) of five days (PAHO 1982), perhaps suggesting that their health status may be better than Peru's (4), but perhaps also that the administration and utilization of hospitals in Peru may be less efficient. If the Peruvian ALOS were reduced to (for instance) five days, most of the country's health regions would have a surplus of beds, and Peru as a whole would have an excess of 17,000 beds.

The excess of beds is smaller if we look solely at MOH facilities (HSA-Peru 1986e:43-45). Only four regions have a substantially larger supply than potential need (Lima, Callao, Ica, and Arequipa) assuming a 10-day ALOS. At the hospital area level, the result of excluding the private sub-sector and IPSS is most evident; the sectorial bed surpluses diminish and the deficits increase. Obviously, if the ALOS in MOH facilities could be shortened to 5 days, the situation would improve; the improvement, however, would not be as significant as for the sector as a whole. This suggests that, with better coordination, some of the public sub-sector's need for beds could be met by private and IPSS facilities.

Evolution of Physical Facilities, 1975-1985

When 1985 data are compared with 1975 data at the departmental level (see Tables 5.7 and 5.8), it is clear that in several cases the maldistribution of health care facilities in Peru has been reduced over the last decade. For example, using the same parameters to calculate the availability of and potential need for hospital beds in 1975 and 1985, there is a surplus of beds in both years. However, the 1975 excess was 62 percent larger than in 1985.

The departments whose deficits have increased or whose surpluses have decreased are La Libertad, Junin, Tumbes, Amazonas, Cuzco, Piura and San Martin. The population per hospital bed ratios increased between 1975 (pop./bed in Table 5.7) and 1985 (Table 5.3) for all departments except Ancash, Puno, Huancavelica and Loreto. The national average rose from 533 to 657 inhabitants per bed, indicating that population growth exceeded the increase in the number of available hospital beds.

Primary health care facilities have increased in number more rapidly than the population as a whole. From 1975 to 1985 there was a 47 percent increase in the number of health centers, and a 73 percent increase in health posts. Three-fourths of the new centers are administered by the MOH. Virtually all the new health posts were built and/or implemented by the Ministry as well. Expansion has been greatest in the departments of Lima/Callao, Huancavelica, Junin, and La Libertad. In the case of Lima/Callao, the construction of many new health posts was a response to heavy migration to the capital and the subsequent emergence of numerous densely-populated marginal urban settlements. However, the analysis presented earlier shows there are still not nearly enough health centers and posts in Peru in general—and in Lima/Callao in particular—to provide uniform coverage for all Peruvians.

Maintenance and Physical Status of Health Care Facilities

Thus far, the distribution of health care facilities in Peru has been analyzed without regard for their equipment inventories or states of repair. There is a general lack of data on this subject. Indeed, there has never been sufficient information on the functional characteristics of facilities, at the sectorial level, to design or sustain a national health facilities maintenance system. Health sector authorities have occasionally attempted to implement nationwide equipment censuses, but due to high costs, a scarcity of specialized personnel, and frequent changes of administration, this still has not been done.

In an attempt to address this problem, a simplified survey on the state of health facilities' buildings, utility systems, and equipment was carried out by an HSA-Peru team in Cuzco and Cajamarca (ANSSA-Peru 1986d). While not comprehensive, this survey yielded enough information to enable the MOH to take some immediate action (5). It provided a simplified inventory of buildings, utility systems, and equipment, and their present state of repair; databases to facilitate periodic updating of this inventory; and global indicators for estimating the costs of repair and preventive maintenance of buildings, utility systems, and equipment.

The survey showed that hospital designations bore no relation to their equipment inventories—nor, in consequence, to the services they could offer. For example, there were hospitals classified as "general" in all the hospital areas surveyed; however, their equipment, sizes and bed counts varied widely. One "general" hospital had 63 units of equipment, while another, also listed as "general," had 379 units.

In all hospitals surveyed, the infrastructure had deteriorated by over 50 percent (ANSSA-Peru 1986d). Deterioration was particularly evident in building walls and in surgery areas; in contrast, administrative offices were in the best repair. In both Cuzco and Cajamarca, the utility systems of the hospitals located in the central hospital areas were acceptable, but for rural hospitals the level of utilities deterioration averaged 10 to 50 percent; some had even greater than 50 percent deterioration. Worst off were the water, electrical, and communications systems in the hospital in Chota; the water and sewage systems in La Convencion; and all utility systems in the Canchis hospital. In both regions only 50 percent of all equipment was working normally and about 17 percent was in complete disrepair. Worst in this respect was the regional hospital at Cuzco, with only 27 percent of its equipment working properly. In Cajamarca, the most deteriorated equipment was sterilization, power-generating, and cooking equipment, and the main reasons for their disrepair were damage, and, to a lesser degree, obsolescence. In Cuzco, the most serious problems were in pediatric, laundry, and x-ray equipment. The main reasons for these problems were also damage and age. The situation for health centers' buildings and equipment was similar to that of hospitals, except that health centers' utility systems were in somewhat better condition.

Important factors contributing to the poor state of equipment at both hospitals and health centers were the lack of replacements and the great diversity of brands. The equipment in almost all Cuzco and Cajamarca hospitals dated from the time these facilities were constructed (an average of 35 years ago). And there was wide variety among brand names for the same types of equipment (most of which was imported); in some instances, each hospital had a different brand of the same type of equipment. Pieces of equipment often remained unused for years, awaiting spare parts from abroad.

With few exceptions, health posts in Cuzco and Cajamarca were rarely built for that purpose; many had been existing buildings donated by the local residents. Yet the overall physical condition of these buildings was fairly acceptable, with the exception of Canchis, where the majority of the posts (80 percent) were in poor condition. However, 75 percent of the health posts in Cajamarca, and 41 percent in Cuzco, had no water or sewage systems. Moreover, 96 percent of the posts in Cajamarca and 66 percent in Cuzco were without electricity. Many posts lacked sterilization and refrigeration equipment—a problem especially serious in the Cuzco facilities. The majority of the health posts surveyed, however, did have the minimum equipment for this type of health facility.

Conclusions

The first priority of any country's Ministry of Health should be to deliver health care equitably, through an efficient referral system, across regions and income groups. Unfortunately, this goal has not yet been achieved in Peru; the structure of existing health care facilities bears little relation to the distribution of the population. Based on the findings described here, a number of important conclusions about the distribution of Peruvian health care facilities emerge.

Health care facilities are heavily concentrated in the major urban areas of Peru. This maldistribution is so severe that even though the raw numbers of health care facilities appear to be adequate for a country of close to 20 million people in 1985, many rural areas of the country are grossly underserved. The concentration of major hospitals in urban coastal areas—particularly in the Lima/Callao area—is especially notable. Eighty-four percent of the hospitals in Peru with 500+ beds are located in metropolitan Lima/Callao. The capital also has 55 percent of all hospital beds, available for only 31 percent of the Peruvian population. While it may be difficult to change the *status quo* the construction of new facilities should not be undertaken without taking existing imbalances into account.

All the hospital areas in Peru have at least one hospital with 30 or more beds, but there is no proportioned array of hospitals throughout all health regions. The MOH runs too many large hospitals and too few medium-sized ones, preventing its network from functioning efficiently and equitably. In some health regions, hospitals of similar size run by the MOH, IPSS, and the private sub-sector exist side by side. This is especially true of Lima/Callao, where there is extreme duplication. The situation calls for better coordination at the sectorial level prior to the construction of new facilities by any of the principal institutional providers of health care. One of the most important conclusions of the study is that an efficient structuring of health care facilities for Peru—the central responsibility of the MOH—can be accomplished only by considering the health sector as a whole.

Health centers and posts are better distributed than hospitals, yet the need for them still exceeds their supply in both rural and urban areas of the country. Specifically, more of these facilities are needed in rural Cajamarca, Lambayeque, Cuzco and Huancayo, as well as in Lima/ Callao—especially in the metropolitan area's outlying residential areas, which are characterized by extreme poverty and rapid population growth.

When the present situation is compared, at the departmental level, with that of ten years ago, it is clear that the overall situation has improved. Although there was a larger excess supply of beds in 1975 than in 1985, there was a greater deficit of health centers and posts, and their distribution, considering demographic density, was more uneven than it is now.

Many Peruvian health care facilities suffer from physical deterioration. Based on information collected in the regions of Cajamarca and Cuzco, water, sewage and electric systems were found to be the most seriously deteriorated, with some health care facilities functioning at less than 50 percent of their capacity due to these problems. Equipment was often as old as the buildings themselves, and repair and maintenance are exceedingly difficult because of the large variety of brands of equipment. Yet many facilities lacked the minimum amount of equipment required to operate properly. The MOH should not only work toward a more equitable distribution of new health care facilities, but should also take immediate steps to repair, maintain, and resupply their existing facilities.

Finally, the need for a modern data-processing system on physical infrastructure, utility systems, and equipment—so that the overall state of each of these can be seen at a glance when administrative decisions need to be made—is evident. A by-product of the research on facilities summarized here was the provision of the basic elements for developing such a system.

Footnotes

1. The HSA-Peru technical document on which the chapter is based (HSA-Peru 1986e) includes a complete set of tables for both departments and health regions.

2. In actual practice, even poor Peruvians often bypass their local health posts or health centers, since these are apt to be understaffed and undersupplied. Many patients also go directly to hospitals because these are likely to be geographically closer.

3. The number of bed-days per year was determined by multiplying the number of available hospital beds by 365. Potential need for bed-days was calculated by multiplying the population size first by 5 percent and then by 10 days. These two figures are based on observations of population behavior across various years, and on ENNSA 1984. The first figure represents the approximately 5 percent of the population of Peru that is hospitalized once a year. (Note that any bed occupancy percentage assumes a health status profile, and that a more reliable analysis would require the use of different percentages

per department or health region/hospital area, considering their diverse health characteristics.) The second figure is the average length of stay per patient (ALOS). All estimates have been made for health regions and hospital areas existing in July 1985.

4. Presumably reflecting a lower incidence of illness and accidents requiring less hospitalization.

5. The main objective of the survey was to generate data that could be used to design a systematic program for maintaining the physical infrastructure of MOH facilities. Using the experience gained in these two case studies, the survey could easily be extended to the rest of the country at relatively low cost.

TABLE 5.1

Distribution and Density of Population by Department, Peru, 1985

Department	Region	Population	Population density (Pop./sq.km.)
Amazonas	J/S	296,700	7.18
Ancash	S/C	907,400	24.75
Apurimac	S	354,900	17.27
Arequipa	S/C	833,200	13.12
Ayacucho	S	543,500	12.30
Cajamarca	S/J	1,157,500	33.14
Cuzco	S	942,700	12.35
Huancavelica	S	368,200	17.47
Huanuco	S/J	546,900	15.82
Ica	C	486,500	22.89
Junin	S/J	988,700	22.79
La Libertad	S/C	1,094,000	47.07
Lambayeque	C	803,500	58.49
Lima/Callao	C	6,246,400	183.89
Loreto	J	574,900	1.51
Madre de Dios	J	41,500	0.53
Moquegua	S/C	116,400	7.41
Pasco	J/S	254,500	10.80
Piura	C/S	1,297,800	35.65
Puno	S	959,100	13.25
San Martin	J	385,500	7.37
Tacna	C	174,300	11.44
Tumbes	C	123,400	26.08
Ucayali	J	200,000	2.04
Total		19,697,500	15.33

Note: S = sierra; C = coast; J = jungle

Sources: INE 1978; INP 1985.

TABLE 5.2

Health Care Facilities in Peru
1985

Department	Health Sector				Ministry of Health				IPSS			
					Hospitals				Hospitals			
	Hosp.	HC	HP	Beds	No.	Beds	HC	HP	No.	Beds	HC	HP
Amazonas	1	14	77	100	1	100	11	64	0	0	1	3
Ancash	21	33	86	845	11	575	31	81	1	140	0	0
Apurimac	2	16	56	185	2	185	11	55	0	0	1	0
Arequipa	23	59	107	1,923	5	1,146	41	68	2	430	10	15
Ayacucho	8	13	93	326	7	317	11	93	0	0	0	0
Cajamarca	4	24	89	161	4	161	24	89	0	0	0	0
Cusco	5	30	126	858	4	840	22	124	0	0	0	1
Huancavelica	7	23	86	198	1	110	21	84	0	0	0	0
Huanuco	7	14	83	418	3	341	10	83	0	0	1	0
Ica	12	24	30	1,076	6	671	23	29	2	266	0	0
Junin	22	37	135	1,303	8	735	37	133	1	149	0	2
La Libertad	17	39	115	1,052	6	439	27	100	2	234	2	3
Lambayeque	18	22	29	1,127	3	325	20	29	1	422	0	0
Lima/Callao	130	221	199	16,449	28	8,060	179	125	7	2,675	6	4
Loreto	10	35	112	754	3	299	13	96	1	56	0	0
Madre de Dios	2	4	14	50	2	50	2	14	0	0	1	0
Moquegua	5	7	26	355	2	191	5	21	0	0	0	2
Pasco	10	17	59	496	2	88	8	59	2	170	6	0
Piura	16	51	94	1,119	3	404	36	93	1	157	2	0
Puno	10	33	121	450	8	407	30	100	1	31	1	3
San Martin	4	34	113	216	4	216	28	109	0	0	0	0
Tacna	1	15	23	256	1	256	10	22	0	0	1	0
Tumbes	1	11	29	92	1	92	6	19	0	0	1	0
Ucayali	2	9	23	175	2	175	6	22	0	0	1	0
Total	338	785	1,925	29,984	117	16,183	612	1,712	21	4,730	34	33

(Continued)

Note: HC = Health Centers
HP= Health Posts

Source: MOH 1985.

TABLE 5.2 (Cont.)

Department	Uniformed Forces				Other Public				Private			
	Hospitals		HC	HP	Hospital		HC	HP	Hospitals		HC	HP
	No.	Beds			No.	Beds			No.	Beds		
Amazonas	0	0	2	10	0	0	0	0	0	0	0	0
Ancash	0	0	0	0	1	12	1	5	8	118	1	0
Apurimac	0	0	4	0	0	0	0	0	0	0	0	1
Arequipa	0	0	3	7	1	35	1	0	15	312	4	17
Ayacucho	0	0	1	0	0	0	1	0	1	9	0	0
Cajamarca	0	0	0	0	0	0	0	0	0	0	0	0
Cusco	0	0	4	0	1	18	0	0	0	0	4	1
Huancavelica	0	0	1	0	0	0	0	0	6	88	1	2
Huanuco	0	0	3	0	0	0	0	0	4	77	0	0
Ica	0	0	1	1	0	0	0	0	4	139	0	0
Junin	1	12	0	0	8	314	0	0	4	93	0	0
La Libertad	0	0	3	0	5	268	7	11	4	111	0	1
Lambayeque	3	86	0	0	6	234	1	0	5	60	1	0
Lima/Callao	6	1,861	11	0	3	198	4	12	86	3,655	21	58
Loreto	2	288	22	16	1	8	0	0	3	103	0	0
Madre de Dios	0	0	1	0	0	0	0	0	0	0	0	0
Moquegua	0	0	2	2	0	0	0	1	3	164	0	0
Pasco	0	0	1	0	1	81	0	0	5	157	2	0
Piura	1	100	11	1	2	160	1	0	9	298	1	0
Puno	1	12	2	2	0	0	0	16	0	0	0	0
San Martin	0	0	5	4	0	0	0	0	0	0	1	0
Tacna	0	0	2	1	0	0	1	0	0	0	1	0
Tumbes	0	0	4	8	0	0	0	2	0	0	0	0
Ucayali	0	0	1	0	0	0	0	0	0	0	1	1
Total	14	2,359	84	52	29	1,328	17	47	157	5,384	38	81

Note: HC = Health Centers
HP = Health Posts

Source: MOH 1985.

TABLE 5.3

Ratios of Population per Unit of Health Care Facility, Health Sector, 1985

Department	Pop./ bed	Pop./ HC	Pop./ HP
Amazonas	2,967	21,193	3,853
Ancash	1,074	27,497	10,551
Apurimac	1,918	22,181	6,338
Arequipa	433	14,122	7,787
Ayacucho	1,667	41,808	5,844
Cajamarca	7,189	48,229	13,006
Cusco	1,099	31,423	7,482
Huancavelica	1,860	16,009	4,281
Huanuco	1,308	39,064	6,589
Ica	452	20,271	16,217
Junin	759	26,722	7,324
La Libertad	1,040	28,051	9,513
Lambayeque	713	36,523	27,707
Lima/Callao	380	28,264	31,389
Loreto	762	16,426	5,133
Madre de Dios	830	10,375	2,964
Moquegua	328	16,629	4,477
Pasco	513	14,971	4,314
Piura	1,160	25,447	13,806
Puno	2,131	29,064	7,926
San Martin	1,785	11,338	3,412
Tacna	681	11,620	7,578
Tumbes	1,341	11,218	4,255
Ucayali	1,143	22,222	8,696
Total	657	25,092	10,232

Sources: TABLES 5.1 and 5.2.

TABLE 5.4

Participation of the Ministry of Health in the Overall Supply of Physical Infrastructure for Health Care, 1985

Department	Hosp.	Beds	Beds as percent of sect. tot.	HC	HC as percent of sect. tot.	HP	HP as percent of sect. tot.
Amazonas	1	100	100.00	11	78.57	64	83.12
Ancash	11	575	68.05	31	93.94	81	94.19
Apurimac	2	185	100.00	11	68.75	55	98.21
Arequipa	5	1,146	59.59	41	69.49	68	63.55
Ayacucho	7	317	97.24	11	84.62	93	100.00
Cajamarca	4	161	100.00	24	100.00	89	100.00
Cusco	4	840	97.90	22	73.33	124	98.41
Huancavelica	1	110	55.56	21	91.30	84	97.67
Huanuco	3	341	81.58	10	71.43	83	100.00
Ica	6	671	62.36	23	95.83	29	96.67
Junin	8	735	56.41	37	100.00	133	98.52
La Libertad	6	439	41.73	27	69.23	100	86.96
Lambayeque	3	325	28.84	20	90.91	29	100.00
Lima/Callao	28	8,060	49.00	179	81.00	125	62.81
Loreto	3	299	39.66	13	37.14	96	85.71
Madre de Dios	2	50	100.00	2	50.00	14	100.00
Moquegua	2	191	53.80	5	71.43	21	80.77
Pasco	2	88	17.74	8	47.06	59	100.00
Piura	3	404	36.10	36	70.59	93	98.94
Puno	8	407	90.44	30	90.91	100	82.64
San Martin	4	216	100.00	28	82.35	109	96.46
Tacna	1	256	100.00	10	66.67	22	95.65
Tumbes	1	92	100.00	6	54.55	19	65.52
Ucayali	2	175	100.00	6	66.67	22	95.65
Total	117	16,183	53.97	612	77.96	1,712	88.94

Sources: TABLES 5.1 and 5.2.

TABLE 5.5

Referral Network of Health Facilities by Hospital Areas and Health Regions
Health Sector, Peru, 1985

Regions	Hospital Areas	Hospitals						HC	HP	Indicators			
		Hosp.	Beds	Type						HP/HC	HC/ pop.den.	HP/ pop.den.	Pop./ Bed
				"1"	"2"	"3"	"4"						
Reg.I	TUMBES	1	92	0	1	0	0	11	29	2.64	0.44	1.15	1,298
PIURA	SULLANA	7	445	4	3	0	0	30	41	1.37	0.50	0.69	2,236
	PIURA (*)	9	674	5	2	2	0	21	53	2.52	0.73	1.84	938
		17	1,211	9	6	2	0	62	123	1.98	1.54	3.05	1,442
Reg. II	LAMBAYEQUE (*)	18	1,127	13	3	1	1	22	33	1.50	0.41	0.62	732
CHICLAYO	JAEN	1	30	1	0	0	0	3	25	8.33	0.12	0.98	8,714
	AMAZONAS	1	100	0	1	0	0	14	74	5.29	2.00	10.56	2,893
		20	1,257	14	4	1	1	39	132	3.38	1.90	6.42	1,094
Reg. III	CHOTA	1	60	0	1	0	0	8	20	2.50	0.18	0.44	5,776
CAJAMARCA	CAJAMARCA (*)	2	71	2	0	0	0	14	46	3.29	0.45	1.48	7,308
		3	131	2	1	0	0	22	66	3.00	0.62	1.86	6,606

(Continued)

TABLE 5.5 (Cont.)

Regions	Hospital Areas	Hospitals								Indicators			
		Hosp.	Beds	Type "1"	Type "2"	Type "3"	Type "4"	HC	HP	HP/HC	HC/ pop.den.	HP/ pop.den.	Pop./ Bed
Reg. IV	PACASMAYO	2	132	1	1	0	0	4	16	4.00	0.07	0.28	897
TRUJILLO	TRUJILLO (*)	14	887	9	4	1	0	32	67	2.09	0.55	1.15	889
	HUAMACHUCO	1	33	1	0	0	0	2	26	13.00	0.09	1.11	4,415
		17	1,052	11	5	1	0	38	109	2.87	0.79	2.26	1,000
Reg. V	CHIMBOTE	10	488	7	2	1	0	12	26	2.17	0.42	0.92	711
HUARAZ	POMABAMBA	1	30	1	0	0	0	4	8	2.00	0.20	0.40	2,549
	HUARAZ (*)	10	327	9	1	0	0	18	52	2.89	0.93	2.69	1,548
		21	845	17	3	1	0	34	86	2.53	1.54	3.91	1,100
Reg. VI	RIMAC (*)	72	12,121	38	15	6	13	108	26	0.24	0.10	0.02	335
LIMA	CHOSICA	13	826	8	4	0	1	49	89	1.82	1.39	2.52	192
	CANETE	3	160	2	1	0	0	11	23	2.09	0.67	1.41	1,125
		88	13,107	48	20	6	14	168	138	0.82	0.73	0.60	336
Reg. VII	CHINCHA	22	1,249	14	8	0	0	6	15	2.50	0.23	0.57	126
ICA	PISCO (*)	12	875	7	3	2	0	23	52	2.26	1.21	2.75	360
	LUCANAS	4	90	4	0	0	0	3	30	10.00	0.46	4.55	2,504
		38	2,214	25	11	2	0	32	97	3.03	2.61	7.91	315

Reg. VIII	CASTILLA	4	75	4	0	0	0	17	20	1.18	4.00	4.70	1,009
AREQUIPA	CAMANA	6	129	5	1	0	0	7	20	2.86	2.02	5.76	473
	AREQUIPA (*)	10	1,319	6	1	2	1	33	59	1.79	1.23	2.19	472
	ISLAY	3	400	1	1	1	0	2	7	3.50	0.20	0.71	123
		23	1,923	12	3	3	1	59	106	1.80	4.64	8.33	420
Reg. IX	MOQUEGUA	5	355	1	4	0	0	7	26	3.71	0.97	3.61	318
TACNA	TACNA (*)	1	256	0	0	1	0	15	23	1.53	1.36	2.09	654
		6	611	1	4	1	0	22	49	2.23	2.43	5.41	459
Reg. X	PUNO (*)	5	287	4	0	1	0	8	48	6.00	0.34	2.04	1,358
PUNO	SAN ROMAN	3	68	2	1	0	0	7	32	4.57	0.32	1.44	4,003
	AZANGARO	1	18	1	0	0	0	6	30	5.00	0.62	3.08	10,249
	MELGAR	1	77	0	1	0	0	12	11	0.92	2.34	2.15	1,304
		10	450	7	2	1	0	33	121	3.67	2.35	8.61	2,104
Reg. XI	CANCHIS	1	65	0	1	0	0	7	25	3.57	0.43	1.52	4,159
CUZCO	MADRE DE DIOS	2	50	2	0	0	0	4	12	3.00	6.18	18.55	699
	CUZCO 1 (*)	1	347	0	0	0	1	11	37	3.36	1.48	4.98	712
	CUZCO 2	2	318	1	0	1	0	11	39	3.55	0.76	2.68	612
	LA CONVENCION	1	128	0	1	0	0	1	33	0.00	0.23	7.49	1,381
	ABANCAY	1	125	0	1	0	0	7	35	5.00	0.59	2.95	1,195
	ANDAHUAYLAS	1	60	0	1	0	0	8	17	2.13	0.28	0.59	2,662
		9	1,093	3	4	1	1	49	198	4.04	6.97	28.16	1,128

(Continued)

TABLE 5.5 (Cont.)

Regions	Hospital Areas	Hospitals								Indicators			
		Hosp.	Beds	Type				HC	HP	HP/HC	HC/ pop.den.	HP/ pop.den.	Pop./ Bed
				"1"	"2"	"3"	"4"						
Reg. XII AYACUCHO	AYACUCHO (*)	5	251	4	1	0	0	11	57	5.18	0.43	2.20	1,846
Reg. XIII HUANCAYO	HUANCAVELICA	4	168	3	1	0	0	8	37	4.63	0.31	1.45	1,082
	HUANCAYO (*)	7	406	5	2	0	0	28	62	2.21	0.58	1.29	1,320
	JAUJA	9	607	6	1	2	0	9	34	3.78	0.29	1.10	330
	TARMA	1	120	0	1	0	0	4	11	2.75	0.11	0.29	966
	SELVA CENTRAL	5	178	4	1	0	0	9	74	8.22	1.47	12.07	1,456
	JUNIN	1	25	1	0	0	0	1	6	6.00	0.07	0.40	1,269
		27	1,504	19	6	2	0	59	224	3.80	3.21	12.20	881
Reg. XIV HUANUCO	PASCO	9	463	5	4	0	0	12	27	2.25	0.42	0.94	398
	HUANUCO (*)	3	195	2	0	1	0	8	30	3.75	0.52	1.95	1,790
	LA UNION	3	80	3	0	0	0	2	31	15.50	0.07	1.01	716
	TINGO MARIA	1	143	0	1	0	0	2	18	9.00	0.09	0.83	665
	PUCALLPA	2	175	1	1	0	0	9	25	2.78	4.75	13.18	1,111
		18	1,056	11	6	1	0	33	131	3.97	5.17	20.53	834

Reg. XV	HUALLAGA	1	27	1	0	0	0	7	23	3.29	1.85	6.08	4,554
MOYOBAMBA	SAN MARTIN	1	135	0	1	0	0	18	73	4.06	1.65	6.70	1,119
	MOYOBAMBA (*)	2	54	2	0	0	0	9	18	2.00	0.55	1.10	1,806
		4	216	3	1	0	0	34	114	3.35	4.79	16.05	1,720
Reg. XVI	YURIMAGUAS	2	64	1	1	0	0	5	26	5.20	3.45	17.94	1,520
IQUITOS	IQUITOS (*)	8	690	3	3	2	0	32	87	2.72	21.64	58.83	670
		10	754	4	4	2	0	37	113	3.05	25.11	76.69	742
Reg. XVII	CHANCAY	11	852	6	3	2	0	24	52	2.17	0.70	1.51	518
CALLAO	CALLAO (*)	11	1,457	9	0	0	2	29	9	0.31	0.01	0.00	304
		22	2,309	15	3	2	2	53	61	1.15	0.78	0.89	383
Totals		338	29,984	209	84	26	19	785	1,925	2.45	53.59	131.42	628

Note: (*) Regional headquarters

Source: MOH 1985.

TABLE 5.6

Supply of and Potential Need for Hospital Beds, Health Sector, 1985

Region	Hospital Areas	Need for beds (10 ALOS) [N1] (**)	Need for beds (5 ALOS) [N2]	Annual supply of beds [S]	N1 - S (10 ALOS)	N2 - S (5 ALOS)	Bed deficit (10 ALOS)	Bed deficit (5 ALOS)
Reg. I	Tumbes	59,700	29,850	33,580	26,120	(3,730)	72	(10)
Piura	Sullana	497,606	248,803	162,425	335,181	86,378	918	237
	Piura (*)	316,051	158,025	246,010	70,041	(87,985)	192	(241)
		873,357	436,678	442,015	431,342	(5,337)	1,182	(15)
Reg. II	Lambayeque (*)	412,412	206,206	411,355	1,057	(205,149)	3	(562)
Chiclayo	Jaen	130,708	65,354	10,950	119,758	54,404	328	149
	Amazonas	144,637	72,318	36,500	108,137	35,818	296	98
		687,756	343,878	458,805	228,951	(114,927)	627	(315)
Reg. III	Chota	173,274	86,637	21,900	151,374	64,737	415	177
Cajamarca	Cajamarca (*)	259,451	129,726	25,915	233,536	103,811	640	284
		432,725	216,362	47,815	384,910	168,547	1,055	462

Reg. IV	Pacasmayo	59,232	29,616	48,180	11,052	(18,564)	30	(51)
Trujillo	Trujillo (*)	394,180	197,090	323,755	70,425	(126,665)	193	(347)
	Huamachuco	72,845	36,423	12,045	60,800	24,378	167	67
		526,256	263,128	383,980	142,276	(120,852)	390	(331)
Reg. V	Chimbote	173,435	86,718	178,120	(4,685)	(91,403)	(13)	(250)
Huaraz	Pomabamba	38,234	19,117	10,950	27,284	8,167	75	22
	Huaraz (*)	253,068	126,534	119,355	133,713	7,179	366	20
		464,736	232,368	308,425	156,311	(76,057)	428	(208)
Reg. VI	Rimac (*)	2,032,845	1,016,422	4,424,165	(2,391,321)	(3,407,743)	(6,552)	(9,336)
Lima	Chosica	79,350	39,675	301,490	(222,140)	(261,815)	(609)	(717)
	Canete	90,021	45,010	58,400	31,621	(13,390)	87	(37)
		2,202,215	1,101,108	4,784,055	(2,581,840)	(3,682,948)	(7,074)	(10,090)
Reg. VII	Chincha	78,424	39,212	455,885	(377,461)	(416,673)	(1,034)	(1,142)
Ica	Pisco (*)	157,524	78,762	319,375	(161,851)	(240,613)	(443)	(659)
	Lucanas	112,667	56,334	32,850	79,817	23,484	219	64
		348,615	174,308	808,110	(459,495)	(633,803)	(1,259)	(1,736)
Reg. VIII	Castilla	37,842	18,921	27,375	10,467	(8,454)	29	(23)
Arequipa	Camana	30,539	15,269	47,085	(16,547)	(31,816)	(45)	(87)
	Arequipa (*)	311,239	155,619	481,435	(170,197)	(325,816)	(466)	(893)
	Islay	24,681	12,341	146,000	(121,319)	(133,660)	(332)	(366)
		404,300	202,150	701,895	(297,595)	(499,745)	(815)	(1,369)

(Continued)

TABLE 5.6 (Cont.)

Region	Hospital Areas	Need for beds (10 ALOS) [N1] (**)	Need for beds (5 ALOS) [N2]	Annual supply of beds [S]	N1 - S (10 ALOS)	N2 - S (5 ALOS)	Bed deficit (10 ALOS)	Bed deficit (5 ALOS)
Reg. IX	Moquegua	56,500	28,250	129,575	(73,075)	(101,325)	(200)	(278)
Tacna	Tacna (*)	83,700	41,850	93,440	(9,740)	(51,590)	(27)	(141)
		140,200	70,100	223,015	(82,815)	(152,915)	(227)	(419)
Reg. X	Puno (*)	194,831	97,415	104,755	90,076	(7,340)	247	(20)
Puno	San Roman	136,096	68,048	24,820	111,276	43,228	305	118
	Azangaro	92,237	46,118	6,570	85,667	39,548	235	108
	Melgar	50,187	25,094	28,105	22,082	(3,012)	60	(8)
		473,350	236,675	164,250	309,100	72,425	847	198
Reg. XI	Canchis	135,175	67,587	23,725	111,450	43,862	305	120
Cuzco	Madre de Dios	17,478	8,739	18,250	(772)	(9,511)	(2)	(26)
	Cuzco 1 (*)	123,481	61,740	126,655	(3,175)	(64,915)	(9)	(178)
	Cuzco 2	97,311	48,656	116,070	(18,759)	(67,415)	(51)	(185)
	La Convencion	88,381	44,191	46,720	41,661	(2,530)	114	(7)
	Abancay	74,707	37,354	45,625	29,082	(8,272)	80	(23)
	Andahuaylas	79,872	39,936	21,900	57,972	18,036	159	49
		616,404	308,202	398,945	217,459	(90,743)	596	(249)

Reg. XII Ayacucho	Ayacucho (*)	231,638	115,819	91,615	140,023	24,204	384	66
Reg. XIII Huancayo	Huancavelica	90,863	45,432	61,320	29,543	(15,889)	81	(44)
	Huancayo (*)	267,999	133,999	148,190	119,809	(14,191)	328	(39)
	Jauja	100,293	50,147	221,555	(121,262)	(171,409)	(332)	(470)
	Tarma	57,965	28,983	43,800	14,165	(14,818)	39	(41)
	Selva Central	129,567	64,783	64,970	64,597	(187)	177	(1)
	Junin	15,863	7,931	9,125	6,738	(1,194)	18	(3)
		662,549	331,274	548,960	113,589	(217,686)	311	(596)
Reg. XIV Huanuco	Pasco	92,176	46,088	168,995	(76,820)	(122,907)	(210)	(337)
	Huanuco (*)	174,571	87,286	71,175	103,396	16,111	283	44
	La Union	28,620	14,310	29,200	(580)	(14,890)	(2)	(41)
	Tingo Maria	47,573	23,787	52,195	(4,622)	(28,409)	(13)	(78)
	Pucallpa	97,200	48,600	63,875	33,325	(15,275)	91	(42)
		440,140	220,070	385,440	54,700	(165,370)	150	(453)
Reg. XV Moyobamba	Huallaga	61,475	30,737	9,855	51,620	20,882	141	57
	San Martin	75,503	37,751	49,275	26,228	(11,524)	72	(32)
	Moyobamba (*)	48,773	24,387	19,710	29,063	4,677	80	13
		185,750	92,875	78,840	106,910	14,035	293	38

(Continued)

TABLE 5.6 (Cont.)

Region	Hospital Areas	Need for beds (10 ALOS) [N1] (**)	Need for beds (5 ALOS) [N2]	Annual supply of beds [S]	N1 - S (10 ALOS)	N2 - S (5 ALOS)	Bed deficit (10 ALOS)	Bed deficit (5 ALOS)
Reg. XVI	Yurimaguas	48,629	24,315	23,360	25,269	955	69	3
Iquitos	Iquitos (*)	231,271	115,636	251,850	(20,579)	(136,215)	(56)	(373)
		279,900	139,950	275,210	4,690	(135,260)	13	(371)
Reg. XVII	Chancay	220,820	110,410	310,980	(90,160)	(200,570)	(247)	(550)
Callao	Callao (*)	221,707	110,853	531,805	(310,099)	(420,952)	(850)	(1,153)
		442,527	221,263	842,785	(400,259)	(621,522)	(1,097)	(1,703)
		9,412,415	4,706,207	10,944,160	(1,531,746)	(6,237,953)	(4,197)	(17,090)

NOTE: Parenthesis indicates SURPLUS

(*) Head of the Region

(**) ALOS = average length of stay

TABLE 5.7

Participation of the Ministry of Health in the Overall Supply of Physical Infrastructure for Health Care, 1975

Department	Health Sector				Sectoral Indicators		
	Hosp.	HC	HP	Beds	Pop./ bed	Pop./ HC	Pop./ HP
Amazonas	3	11	71	143	1,428	18,555	2,875
Ancash	19	24	57	746	1,129	35,083	14,772
Apurimac	2	6	36	190	1,837	58,183	9,697
Arequipa	22	37	65	1,989	300	16,103	9,166
Ayacucho	8	8	62	339	1,493	63,263	8,163
Cajamarca	4	20	49	238	4,888	58,170	23,743
Cusco	6	20	84	910	916	41,670	9,921
Huancavelica	3	4	24	151	2,668	100,700	16,783
Huanuco	5	7	55	410	1,192	69,814	8,885
Ica	17	19	26	1,158	374	22,816	16,673
Junin	20	19	58	1,323	614	42,753	14,005
La Libertad	21	34	53	1,614	562	26,697	17,126
Lambayeque	17	23	42	811	712	25,122	13,757
Lima y Callao	136	188	32	15,889	272	22,949	134,825
Loreto	4	9	76	570	1,068	67,633	8,009
Madre de Dios	2	3	10	45	676	10,133	3,040
Moquegua	4	7	14	258	308	11,357	5,679
Pasco	9	10	19	464	468	21,720	11,432
Piura	15	33	70	1,082	1,001	32,818	15,471
Puno	8	20	80	421	2,217	46,665	11,666
San Martin	5	8	80	206	1,314	33,838	3,384
Tacna	2	7	12	413	272	16,029	9,350
Tumbes	2	11	8	164	626	9,336	12,838
Ucayali	3	5	27	221	905	40,000	7,407
TOTAL	337	533	1,110	29,755	533	29,773	14,296

(Continued)

TABLE 5.7 (Cont.)

Department	Ministry of Health						
	Hosp. sect. tot.	Beds	Beds as percent of	HC	HC as percent of sect. tot.	HP	HP as percent of sect. tot.
Amazonas	3	143	100.00	9	81.82	71	100.00
Ancash	10	507	67.96	22	91.67	47	82.46
Apurimac	2	190	100.00	6	100.00	36	100.00
Arequipa	5	1294	65.06	19	51.35	55	84.62
Ayacucho	5	304	89.68	6	75.00	62	100.00
Cajamarca	3	228	95.80	18	90.00	49	100.00
Cusco	4	874	96.04	17	85.00	84	100.00
Huancavelica	1	109	72.19	2	50.00	24	100.00
Huanuco	3	350	85.37	7	100.00	55	100.00
Ica	6	723	62.44	11	57.89	26	100.00
Junin	7	772	58.35	10	52.63	58	100.00
La Libertad	8	954	59.11	22	64.71	28	52.83
Lambayeque	3	275	33.91	17	73.91	17	40.48
Lima y Callao	27	7422	46.71	104	55.32	28	87.50
Loreto	2	230	40.35	7	77.78	49	64.47
Madre de Dios	2	45	100.00	2	66.67	10	100.00
Moquegua	2	160	62.02	4	57.14	14	100.00
Pasco	1	60	12.93	6	60.00	19	100.00
Piura	4	538	49.72	24	72.73	68	97.14
Puno	5	387	91.92	14	70.00	67	83.75
San Martin	4	196	95.15	7	87.50	80	100.00
Tacna	1	343	83.05	5	71.43	12	100.00
Tumbes	1	124	75.61	4	36.36	8	100.00
Ucayali	1	130	58.82	4	80.00	27	100.00
TOTAL	110	16,358	54.98	347	65.10	994	89.55

Sources MOH 1975; INE 1985a.

TABLE 5.8

Comparison of Availability of Hospital Beds in the Health Sector in 1975 and 1985

Department	Population 75	Potential need 75	Supply of beds 75	Deficit 75 (*)	Population 85	Potential need 85	Supply of beds 85	Deficit 85 (*)	Net Change in Deficit (percent) (**)
Amazonas	204,100	102,050	52,195	137	296,700	148,350	36,500	306	124.35
Ancash	842,000	421,000	272,290	407	907,400	453,700	308,425	398	(2.31)
Apurimac	349,100	174,550	69,350	288	354,900	177,450	67,525	301	4.49
Arequipa	595,800	297,900	725,985	(1,173)	833,200	416,600	701,895	(782)	(33.36)
Ayacucho	506,100	253,050	123,735	354	543,500	271,750	118,990	419	18.13
Cajamarca	1,163,400	581,700	86,870	1,356	1,157,500	578,750	58,765	1,425	5.08
Cusco	833,400	416,700	332,150	232	942,700	471,350	313,170	433	87.08
Huancavelica	402,800	201,400	55,115	401	368,200	184,100	72,270	306	(23.55)
Huanuco	488,700	244,350	149,650	259	546,900	273,450	152,570	331	27.65
Ica	433,500	216,750	422,670	(564)	486,500	243,250	392,740	(410)	(27.40)
Junin	812,300	406,150	482,895	(210)	988,700	494,350	475,595	51	(124.44)
La Libertad	907,700	453,850	589,110	(371)	1,094,000	547,000	383,980	447	(220.52)
Lambayeque	577,800	288,900	296,015	(19)	803,500	401,750	411,355	(26)	35.00
Lima y Callao	4,314,400	2,157,200	5,799,485	(9,979)	6,246,400	3,123,200	6,003,885	(7,892)	(20.91)
Loreto	608,700	304,350	208,050	264	574,900	287,450	275,210	34	(87.29)
Madre de Dios	30,400	15,200	16,425	(3)	41,500	20,750	18,250	7	(304.08)
Moquegua	79,500	39,750	94,170	(149)	116,400	58,200	129,575	(196)	31.16
Pasco	217,200	108,600	169,360	(166)	254,500	127,250	181,040	(147)	(11.47)

(Continued)

TABLE 5.8 (Cont.)

Department	Population 75	Potential need 75	Supply of beds 75	Deficit 75 (*)	Population 85	Potential need 85	Supply of beds 85	Deficit 85 (*)	Net Change in Deficit (percent) (**)
Piura	1,083,000	541,500	394,930	402	1,297,800	648,900	408,435	659	64.06
Puno	933,300	466,650	153,665	857	959,100	479,550	164,250	864	0.74
San Martin	270,700	135,350	75,190	165	385,500	192,750	78,840	312	89.35
Tacna	112,200	56,100	150,745	(259)	174,300	87,150	93,440	(17)	(93.35)
Tumbes	102,700	51,350	59,860	(23)	123,400	61,700	33,580	77	(430.43)
Ucayali	200,000	100,000	80,665	53	200,000	100,000	63,875	99	86.84
Totals	15,868,800	7,934,400	10,860,575	(8,017)	19,697,500	9,848,750	10,944,160	(3,001)	(62.57)

Note: (*) Parenthesis indicates *surplus.*
(**) Parenthesis indicates reduction of the deficit or of the surplus, and all negative values above 100 show a change from surplus to deficit

Sources: Office of Statistics and Information, Ministry of Health.
Health Regions, Ministry of Health.
Projections on Population by Departaments, INE 1985a.

6

Medical Doctors: Determinants of Location

Luis Locay

Of major concern to health care policy-makers in Peru are differences in accessibility to health care services across regions and income groups. One obvious way to reduce these disparities would be to change the existing distribution, both geographical and subsectorial, of some or all types of health care workers. Knowledge of these workers' locations and subsectorial affiliations—Ministry of Health (MOH), Social Security Institute (IPSS), or private sector—are essential to policy decisions aimed at altering the locational and affiliational choices of health care workers. Yet prior to the HSA-Peru this basic information apparently did not exist at a more precise level than that of departments, and the data that did exist for departments appeared to incorporate systematic biases.

An important aim of the HSA-Peru was to provide a more reliable and detailed description than was currently available of the locations and subsectorial affiliations of primary health workers—doctors, nurses, pharmacists, and paramedics. A related aim was to develop a behavioral model of locational decisions for doctors that would clarify the consequences of current and future health sector policies and help to assess the desirability of such policies.

The health sector policy questions that can be addressed in Peru are limited by the kinds of data available. The HSA-Peru study of health care professionals focused on the relative impact on locational decisions of doctors' places of birth and places of study (variables that can be affected by policy-makers via the allocation of resources to medical schools and medical school admissions policies), because data on these variables were available. Doctors' salaries are also an important variable influencing location, but because adequate information on income was unavailable in Peru we did not measure the monetary compensation necessary to induce doctors to practice in particular locations. Neither were we able to estimate the relative importance of unobservable, idiosyncratic factors—such as non-economic personal preferences and contacts—on locational choices (1).

Data and Methods

This analysis is based on two datasets. The first was the 1981 Peruvian census (INE 1981), providing information on occupation, which was supplied on tape by the National Institute of Statistics (INE). While this dataset offers a fairly complete listing of all Peruvian medical practitioners and includes some socioeconomic, demographic, and geographical information as well, the data were already four years old at the time of the study in 1985. Moreover, the census does not identify the subsectors in which individuals work, nor does it provide information on dates and places of study. For these reasons a new dataset on doctors, nurses, and pharmacists was constructed by the HSA-Peru using more up-to-date sources. This dataset is based on a stratified random sample of doctors drawn from the registration of the Peruvian Medical Association (*Colegio Médico*), but also contains more accurate locational data supplied by the MOH, IPSS, and recent voter registration lists. In this chapter we consider only the data on medical doctors, but additional cleaned data are available (ANSSA-Peru 1986e) so that similar studies can be carried out for nurses and perhaps for pharmacists as well.

It has long been recognized that doctors in Peru are heavily concentrated in Lima and Callao. In recent years, confirmation of this has come from the registration records of the *Colegio Médico*, whose widely-quoted figures were used, for example, by Bustios (1985) and the *Mapa de Salud* (Banco Central 1984). Since doctors are required to register with the *Colegio* to practice medicine in Peru, virtually every practicing physician in the country should be registered. Physicians' deaths also appear to be well recorded, since notification of death is necessary prior to the collection of life insurance benefits. The total number of doctors registered with the *Colegio*, therefore, should accurately represent all persons practicing medicine in Peru as well as a few who practice abroad.

The *Colegio's* data on the location of doctors, however, are more suspect. New doctors tend to register immediately with the *Colegio* in Lima if they graduate from medical school there, even though they do not yet have permanent work. Many eventually obtain work in departments other than Lima, and some probably do not update their addresses with the *Colegio*, since there is no penalty for not doing so. We suspect, therefore, that the estimate of the number of doctors working and living in Lima is inflated, and that a similar situation, albeit on a smaller scale, may exist for the three other Peruvian departments with medical schools (Arequipa, Ica, and La Libertad).

These suspicions are confirmed by comparing the distribution figures for the *Colegio* and the census (Table 6.1). While the *Colegio's* registration figures indicate that 72.9 percent of the medical doctors in Peru live in Lima/Callao, the census indicates that only 67.9 percent do. The difference is scattered throughout Peru. For the group of departments (other than Lima) with medical schools, there is little difference between the two figures, while for departments with no medical school the *Colegio's* figure is significantly lower, and probably understated. Therefore, in addition to the *Colegio* records, our second dataset incorporates more accurate locational data.

As Tables 6.1 and 6.2 show, there is a much closer correspondence between our sample and the census in estimating the percentage of doctors in Lima. Indeed, if one compares percentages, the census and the sample are quite similar overall. The considerable differences across departments, especially those with few doctors, result from the fact that the sample was not designed to measure the number of doctors in each department accurately. In addition, the sample contains more women relative to men, a smaller proportion of very young doctors (25-30 years of age), a greater proportion in the 31-40 age group, and a smaller proportion currently living in the departments of their birth. Some of these discrepancies probably reflect long-term changes in the population of doctors underway since 1981 or earlier; one would not be surprised to find, for example, that recently-graduated classes included a higher proportion of women than earlier classes. Others may be accounted for by the sample's greater proportions of recent graduates, which may explain the lower proportion of doctors living in the departments of their birth.

In describing the distribution of Peruvian doctors, we do not rely on a grouping by departments—the only grouping possible using the *Colegio's* figures. Instead, we combine provinces (2) in order to compare those that make up the Lima/Callao metropolitan region with the remaining ones, grouped according to whether or not they contain department capitals, medical schools, or hospitals—important differences that might be expected to affect physicians' locational choices. Using this method, the results (in percentages) are again very close to those of the census (Table 6.2). For 1981, the percentage of the population in each of the provincial groupings is as follows: Lima/Callao, 27.1 percent; provinces containing department capitals other than Lima, with medical schools, 6.5 percent (3); other provinces (besides Lima) containing department capitals, 18.3 percent; provinces without department capitals but with at least one hospital, 31.5 percent; and provinces without hospitals, 16.6 percent. A comparison of the distribution of doctors in relation to population by this grouping reveals a very pronounced skewing of the distribution toward provinces with medical schools and hospitals. Departmental totals significantly obscure this inequality.

The theoretical and empirical work that follows divides the problem of doctor location into three analytic components. The first of these is subsectorial affiliation, with the MOH, IPSS, and the private sector (which for our purposes consists of all doctors not working for the MOH or IPSS) as the possible affiliations. The second is geographical region. Each doctor is located within one of six groups of provinces: *Selva* (jungle), North *Sierra*, South *Sierra*, North Coast, South Coast, and the coastal provinces of Lima and Callao (4). The third analytical component is the province of location.

Subsectorial and Geographical Distribution of Doctors

Table 6.3 shows the distribution of doctors by subsectorial affiliation, for those doctors whose current location could be determined; those for whom information was lacking were excluded, so only percentages are meaningful for comparisons. An estimated 15.8 percent of doctors work for IPSS and 27.3 percent work for the MOH. These numbers are slightly below the historical percentages for the two subsectors. Although the percentages of doctors working in these two branches of the public sector may in fact have fallen in 1985, this lower estimate may also result from the way the study identified current location: if, due to a spelling or coding error, our computer search for matching names missed a doctor working for IPSS or the Ministry, he or she (if identified in voter registration records) was automatically assigned to the private sector.

The dataset used to develop our model (see below) omits doctors for whom information was incomplete, which leaves a subsample of 1,370 doctors. Some of the characteristics of this subsample are described in Tables 6.4 through 6.8, which show the percentages of doctors within the various categories in the subsample. The reader should bear in mind that the sample was not designed to estimate categories containing few doctors accurately.

Table 6.4 presents the number of doctors by affiliation and by region, the first two of our three analytical components. It is evident that IPSS doctors are relatively concentrated in the *Sierra* and the North Coast, and relatively rare in the *Selva* and the South Coast. MOH doctors are heavily concentrated in the Lima area and the South Coast, while private sector doctors are concentrated in the *Sierra* and are relatively scarce in the North *Sierra*.

One potentially important determinant of the geographical location of medical doctors is birthplace. Table 6.5 shows that a higher percentage of private sector doctors practice medicine near their birthplaces (province or region) than either IPSS or MOH doctors. Perhaps being in private practice permits greater flexibility to locate near relatives. Alternatively, it may be that doctors without permanent work who fall into the private sector category by default are more likely to be living with or near their families—*i.e.*, in their birthplaces.

Another potentially important determinant of location is place of study. Table 6.6 shows the distribution of doctors by place of study and institutional affiliation. The most notable feature of this table is the close correspondence between the percentage of doctors trained in Lima (around 70 percent of all Peruvian doctors across all three subsectors) and the percentage currently living there (66 percent of our 1985 sample). Also of possible significance is the relatively large percentage of IPSS doctors trained abroad (almost 16 percent)—a finding that is consistent with their reputation as an elite group.

Table 6.7 shows the percentages of doctors in the three subsectors who are currently living and working in the same regions in which they received their medical educations. As with place of birth, place of study clearly has a strong positive correlation with location, with a higher percentage of private sector doctors than IPSS or MOH doctors practicing medicine in the region where they received their training. The same explanations offered above for place of birth may apply here.

Finally, Table 6.8 shows the distribution of doctors per 10,000 inhabitants according to the degree of electrification of the various provinces (6). Since electrification is an indicator of urbanization and wealth, it should be positively related to the ratio of doctors per inhabitant. Table 6.8 shows that doctors do tend to locate in urbanized areas, and also that IPSS doctors are rare in provinces with less than 50 percent electrification and relatively over-represented in provinces with intermediate levels of electrification (50 to 75 percent). This result is consistent with the provincial grouping results presented in Table 6.2.

Using the Model: Simulations and Policy Questions

Our description of the population of Peruvian doctors, the most complete for Peru since Hall's work in the 1960s, shows that doctors tend to locate in urbanized, higher-income areas, near medical schools and hospitals, near their places of birth, and near where they received their medical degrees. It does not, however, suggest the relative importance of these factors in determining the observed distribution of doctors, or how the factors interact with institutional affiliation, amount of work experience, or gender. The following sections analyze and quantify the effects of all of these factors, in order to develop a behavioral model of doctors' locational choices.

All persons—including doctors—face career choices throughout their lives. The choices we focus on here are those affecting the institutional affiliation and geographical location of individual doctors (7). A doctor newly graduated from medical school and without work at his current location must choose whether to stay or to look for work in another location. Sometimes the choice appears obvious: if an unemployed doctor is offered a good job with IPSS in a large city close to his family, no scientific analysis is needed to explain his acceptance of the offer. However, doctors' choices in Peru are rarely so clear-cut. Instead, they are likely to involve a weighing of conflicting factors, positive and negative. Estimating the comparative force of each factor should help policy-makers to take them properly into account in making their own larger decisions affecting the training and recruitment of doctors.

The observable factors included in our analysis (8) can be classified into three types. Some factors affecting locational choice may be attributes of the individual. The factors included in this group were gender and work experience (expressed as the number of years since graduation from medical school). Other factors differ across locations, but not across individuals. Among these we included the degree of electrification of provinces in 1981, provincial population, and the presence or absence of medical faculties in particular provinces or regions. The third type of factor differs across both locations and individuals. The factors of this type we included were whether an individual had been born in a given province, whether he or she had been born in a given region, and whether he or she had studied there (9).

Presenting the specific statistical model used would be less useful for present purposes than looking at some simulations based on the equations of the model (10). This will provide the reader with a feel for the magnitudes of the various effects observed.

Most of the variables used in the model are not subject to control by health sector policy-makers, who have little influence over such matters as population distribution or the degree of electrification of particular areas. There are a number of ways, however, in which the model can be useful to policy-makers. By illuminating the relationship of the variables to doctors' locational decisions, it may enable public institutions to pursue more effective hiring and promotion practices. Is IPSS aware, for example, of the strong relationship between place of study and the geographical location of its doctors? The model can also be of use to policy-makers by providing quantitative measures of the consequences of those variables they *can* manipulate or influence, such as the admissions policies of medical schools and the allocation of resources. For example, if policy-makers wish to increase the number of doctors in a given region outside of Lima, the model can offer guidance on the consequences of admitting students from that region to Lima medical schools versus training physicians from all over the country in that region. Below, we use the model to project hypothetical distributions of doctors by geographical location or subsectorial affiliation for selected ranges of factors.

Work Experience

The effect of an individual's work experience on his or her locational decisions varies subsectorially. Table 6.9 shows the projected percentages of male doctors born and educated in Lima or Arequipa and working in each of the three subsectors. (The province of Arequipa, located in the South *Sierra*, contains the second largest city in Peru and has a medical school.) The percentage of doctors from Arequipa working for IPSS, for example, substantially increases with experience initially, but then declines. It is also evident from Table 6.9 that doctors from Arequipa are much more likely than doctors from Lima to work in the public sector at every level of work experience.

Table 6.10 shows the projected distribution of male doctors, born and educated in Arequipa and working in each subsector, by location in each of six regions over their working years. As experience increases, the likelihood of doctors who work for the MOH locating in Lima rises significantly. This effect is small for private sector doctors, and does not exist for IPSS doctors.

Table 6.11 shows the likelihood that doctors from Arequipa, throughout their working years, will locate in various types of provinces—if they remain in the South *Sierra*. Once again, the pattern for the MOH is quite different from that of the other two subsectors. If they work for IPSS or in the private sector, Arequipeños are much more likely to locate in Arequipa as they age. The pattern is reversed for the Ministry.

Place of Study

Table 6.12 shows the distribution of male doctors from Arequipa, with 11-15 years of experience and who studied in Lima, by subsectorial affiliation and by region. A comparison of this table with the third columns of Tables 6.9 and 6.10 shows some strong effects of place of study. Doctors from Arequipa have a substantially stronger likelihood of working for the MOH or in the private sector if they studied in Lima than if they studied in Arequipa. Furthermore, if they worked for IPSS or in the private sector they are much less likely to locate in the South *Sierra* and more likely to locate in Lima if they studied in Lima. Region of study is not important for male doctors in the MOH with more than 10 years of experience. The percentage of doctors from Arequipa with ten or more years of experience, who studied in Arequipa and located in the South *Sierra*, can be computed from Tables 6.9 and 6.10 to be 79 percent. The projected percentage who located in Lima is only 8 percent. On the other hand, for doctors who studied in Lima, the corresponding percentages are 59 percent and 19 percent, respectively. In either case, the effect of place of study is substantial.

Policy-makers may be more interested in targeting certain areas within regions than whole regions. Peruvian officials might wish, for example, to increase the number of doctors in the provinces of the South *Sierra* without department capitals. Again, we can compare the effect on choice of province of studying in Lima vs. Arequipa. For doctors who studied in Arequipa, the projected percentage who will locate in a province in the South *Sierra* that does not contain a department capital is 3.9 percent. Interestingly, for those who studied in Lima, that percentage rises slightly to 4.5 percent. This anomalous result—that doctors schooled in a cosmopolitan city would be more likely to move to a provincial town than doctors schooled in Arequipa—is explained by the fact that studying in Lima increases the likelihood of Arequipeños working for the MOH or in the private sector—subsectors whose doctors have a higher propensity for locating in less urban provinces.

Place of Birth

For the next simulation, we hold place of study constant and look at the effect of place of birth. Table 6.13 shows the projected subsectorial distribution of doctors who have 11-15 years of experience, and who studied in Lima, for four birthplaces. Iquitos and Canas were chosen to provide contrast with Lima and Arequipa. Iquitos contains the largest city in the *Selva*; in Canas, in the South *Sierra*, only two percent of homes had electricity in 1981.

Note that *Selva* doctors are very unlikely to work for IPSS. Doctors from relatively remote and less urbanized provinces, such as Canas, are less likely to work for IPSS than similar individuals from more urbanized provinces within the same region, such as Arequipa. Natives of Lima are most likely to work in the private sector.

Table 6.14 shows the distribution of doctors with 11-15 years of experience by birthplace, subsectorial affiliation, and region. The effect of place of birth on choice of region is very significant. Doctors who were born in Arequipa and who work for the MOH, for example, are seven times more likely to locate in the South *Sierra* than similar individuals born in Lima. The effect is even greater for IPSS and private sector doctors. It is interesting to note that the likelihood of locating in the South *Sierra* is substantially lower for natives of Canas than for Arequipeños. This is especially pronounced for IPSS doctors, emphasizing that their locational decisions are very sensitive to urbanization. This result is to be expected, since the users of IPSS services are probably concentrated in urban areas.

As previously noted, shifting doctors from Lima to the South *Sierra* may be of less concern than shifting them to the less urbanized provinces of that region (or others). Table 6.15 shows the distribution of doctors with 11-15 years of experience by provinces (with and without department capitals) in the South *Sierra*, by affiliation and place of birth. It shows that if they practice in the South *Sierra*, natives of Canas have a higher likelihood of locating in provinces there that do not contain department capitals than natives of Arequipa do. This higher likelihood more than compensates for the fact that natives of Canas are less likely to practice in the South *Sierra*, so that for each affiliation, natives of Canas are more likely to locate in provinces in the South *Sierra* without department capitals than are natives of Arequipa. From Tables 6.13 and 6.15 we can compute that 4.5 percent of Arequipeños will locate in provinces in the South *Sierra* that do not contain department capitals. In contrast, 12 percent of natives of Canas will locate in these provinces.

Place of Study vs. Place of Birth

Policy-makers may well wish to know how establishing a new medical school in a region previously without one will affect the distribution of doctors, as compared to changing admissions policies or other alternatives. Since our model measures the effects of medical school location via observations of graduates (who obviously do not exist for hypothetical institutions), we cannot answer this question.

However, we can answer a related question, of interest in its own right, that will give us some guidance. This question concerns the impact on locational choices of directing resources to one medical school or another. Suppose Peruvian policy-makers wish to increase the number of doctors in the South *Sierra*, regardless of their institutional affiliation. Of the policy tools at our disposal, we will confine ourselves to the allocation of resources among medical schools. For simplicity, we will assume that only two schools are being considered, one in Arequipa and one in Lima. In which of these schools should resources be invested for the education of a medical student from Arequipa? If Lima can produce doctors at lower cost than Arequipa, we may be able to get more doctors in the South *Sierra* for the same level of overall expenditure by producing doctors in Lima rather than in Arequipa.

To answer this question, we need to know the likelihood of a native of Arequipa locating in the South *Sierra*, and marginal cost information on medical schools. The latter consideration was beyond the scope of this project, but the former can be estimated from the inferences already presented. For simplicity, let us use the locational choices of doctors with 11 to 15 years of experience, calculated above. Almost 60 percent of Arequipeños who have studied in Lima will locate in the South *Sierra*. The corresponding percentage, if they had studied in Arequipa, is 79 percent. Among natives of Arequipa, an admission to medical school in Lima is only three-fourths as likely to produce an additional South *Sierra* doctor as an admission to a medical school in Arequipa. By considering this together with the costs of educating doctors in the two schools, policy-makers should be able to determine the most efficient way to introduce more physicians into the South *Sierra*.

Returning to the hypothesis that health sector authorities might be more specifically interested in increasing the number of doctors in South *Sierra* provinces without department capitals, we have already seen that Arequipeños have a smaller likelihood of locating in one of those provinces if they studied in Arequipa than if they studied in Lima. Educating such doctors in the South *Sierra* will not increase the likelihood that they will locate in those provinces. Even for natives of Canas who study in Lima, 12 percent will locate in a province of the South *Sierra* without a departmental capital. If they study in Arequipa, the percentage is only slightly better (14 percent). Place of birth makes more difference than place of study in physicians' decisions to locate in a non-capital province.

Gender Differences

Thus far, we have proceeded as if all Peruvian physicians were men. In fact, as Table 6.2 shows, men constitute the overwhelming majority of doctors, but women are an increasing part of this population, and the model disclosed some significant differences in the effects of the variables on women's locational decisions. Table 6.16 shows the simulation results for female doctors from Arequipa who studied in Lima. Comparison with the results for similar males in Table 6.12 shows that women have a greater likelihood than men of working for the MOH (41 percent vs. 36 percent) and a smaller likelihood of working in the private sector (35 percent vs. 40 percent). The likelihood of working for IPSS is about the same for men and women.

These differences are small in comparison to the gender differences in choice of province. Female doctors from Arequipa, if they work for IPSS, are more than three times as likely as their male counterparts to locate in Lima, and about twice as likely to locate there if they work for the MOH. Interestingly, these sharp gender differences do not occur in the private sector, for reasons that are unclear.

If we consider female doctors from Arequipa who also received their medical training in Arequipa, we obtain strikingly different results, as shown by comparing Tables 6.16 and 6.17. Female doctors who studied in Arequipa are far less likely to locate in Lima than if they studied in Lima. This result implies that preferential treatment of women in admission to medical schools outside of Lima, and preferential treatment of men in admission to medical schools in Lima, would be effective in shifting doctors out of Lima (11). A possible explanation for this interesting result is that female doctors, while in medical school or shortly thereafter, tend to marry men who reside in that general area. Since couples are probably more likely to locate near the husband's place of work than the wife's, this could explain the observed relationship, but this hypothesis has not yet been tested.

Urbanization

Our simulations conclude with a brief look at the effect of electrification, a measure of urbanization and wealth, on locational choices. Once again we consider male doctors from Arequipa, whom we assume to have received their medical training in Arequipa. Table 6.18 shows the distribution of these doctors, practicing in the North Coast (12), by subsectorial affiliation and the degree of electrification of the provinces in which they practice. Because electrification may be related to other factors affecting location, notably population, Table 6.18 also shows the fraction of the population of the North Coast in each of the categories (column 4) as well as the ratio of the percentage of doctors to the percentage of population in columns 5, 6, and 7.

The distribution of doctors working for IPSS and the private sector is very similar. It is clear that doctors working for the MOH would be much more likely to be located in a province with low electrification than doctors working for IPSS or in the private sector. The effect of electrification on location is best seen in columns 5 through 7 of Table 6.18, which give a measure of the concentration of doctors relative to population in each group of provinces. As can be seen, the ratio of doctors to inhabitants rises with electrification, with very sharp increases at low levels of electrification.

Summary and Conclusions

This chapter provides a reasonably current description of Peru's population of medical doctors, their institutional affiliations, their geographical distribution, and their social-demographic characteristics. It also presents the results of a behavioral model of subsectorial and geographical locational choice. The work is based in some measure on an existing dataset (INE 1981), but depends primarily on a large sample of current health care workers constructed especially for the HSA-Peru project. This new data source is available for future research into other health care professions (ANSSA-Peru 1986e).

The model was designed under certain constraints imposed by the collective data. It does not address, much less answer, all questions concerning doctors' institutional and locational choices that might be of interest to policy-makers. It does, however, provide systematic information on a number of questions about which only casual observations had previously existed. Based on the findings described here, a number of potentially important conclusions about the distribution of Peruvian doctors emerge.

First, doctors tend to locate in areas near their birthplaces, in their places of medical schooling, and in urban areas, although these tendencies vary in intensity with age and sex. We have not been able to measure the monetary compensation needed to overcome these factors, but our results suggest that it is probably quite high. Inducing many more doctors to locate in impoverished rural locations is not likely to prove a cost-effective method of improving the delivery of health services to those areas. Reliance on systems that place greater emphasis on other health care personnel should prove more fruitful.

Second, about three-fourths of the effect on the probability of locating outside Lima because of place of birth or study can be accounted for by place of birth alone. This finding suggests that if Lima schools have some marginal cost advantage over other medical schools, it may be possible to achieve cost savings without reducing the number of doctors outside Lima.

Third, female doctors have a very strong attachment to place of study. Accordingly, shifting female medical students from Lima to other regions, and shifting male students to Lima, would help to increase the proportion of doctors outside of Lima.

Finally, if a long range goal is not simply to shift doctors out of Lima but to increase their numbers in poorer, less urbanized areas, then place of birth is important. Getting qualified students from targeted areas may be difficult, and this is perhaps an argument for locating any additional medical schools in populous regions where none currently exist.

Footnotes

1. Previous work on health care workers in Peru is quite limited. The most complete is Hall (1969).

2. Departments in Peru are divided into provinces, in one of which—in every department—the departmental capital is located.

3. Since several new medical schools in Peru have yet to graduate their first doctors, this figure refers only to medical schools that have been in existence long enough to have produced doctors.

4. These do not correspond exactly to similar regions defined by INE. See HSA-Peru 1986f:39 for list of provinces that constitute each region.

5. Since there are a substantial number of missing cases, the total number of doctors in each category is underestimated. The relative magnitudes, however, should remain unbiased. We therefore express our results in percentages.

6. Population and electrification figures for each province were derived from the 1981 census (INE 1981).

7. We use the term "choice" in a stricter sense than is used in common discourse. We see an individual as making choices even when he or she is making no career changes, but is choosing instead to follow a course previously chosen. In this sense, alternate choices, even though they may not be attractive, are always available.

8. A fundamental difference among factors that affect locational choices is whether or not the attributes or characteristics of factors are observable by the researcher. A new doctor may decide to locate in a particular area because his uncle, who is also a doctor, owns a clinic there and has offered him a job. While such unobservable, idiosyncratic factors may be the most important ones from the point of view of the individual, from the point of view of statistical behavioral analysis they are a nuisance, introducing "noise" into the relationship between observable factors and locational decisions. Nonetheless, it is important to keep the existence of idiosyncratic factors in mind lest we mistakenly aspire to predict the behavior of any one individual rather than that of groups of individuals of given types.

9. The variables selected for this analysis should not be considered the ideal set. Construction of the model was limited to those variables accessible within the limitations of the available data. We would have liked, for instance, to have identified precisely the communities among which individual doctors choose, but in the face of diverse and unmeasurable individual definitions of these communities, it proved practicable to treat only choices among provinces.

10. The reader is referred to HSA-Peru 1986f for details of the statistical procedures used.

11. This also suggests why nurses, a predominantly female group whose schools are more widely distributed across the country, are much less concentrated in Lima than doctors.

12. We chose a North Coast location for Arequipeños to discount the effects of nativity and place of study, and because that region offered a variety of levels of electrification by province.

TABLE 6.1

Distribution of Doctors by Department

	Colegio 1981		Census 1981 *		1985 Sample *	
Departments	Numbers	Percent	Numbers	Percent	Numbers	Percent
Amazonas	10	0.074	36	0.294	0	0.000
Ancash	160	1.182	201	1.643	290	2.124
Apurimac	11	0.081	26	0.212	73	0.535
Arequipa	723	5.339	661	5.402	989	7.244
Ayacucho	30	0.222	53	0.433	24	0.176
Cajamarca	58	0.428	87	0.711	66	0.483
Cuzco	141	1.041	151	1.234	150	1.099
Huancavelica	12	0.089	21	0.172	33	0.242
Huanuco	86	0.635	59	0.482	74	0.542
Ica	377	2.784	384	3.138	333	2.439
Junin	212	1.565	266	2.174	291	2.131
La Libertad	657	4.852	647	5.287	878	6.431
Lambayeque	359	2.651	365	2.983	378	2.769
Lima, Callao	9871	72.892	8313	67.933	9028	66.125
Loreto, Ucayali	150	1.108	157	1.283	287	2.102
Madre de Dios	9	0.066	18	0.147	2	0.015
Moquegua	94	0.694	84	0.686	45	0.330
Pasco	80	0.591	48	0.392	74	0.542
Piura	302	2.230	356	2.909	305	2.234
Puno	70	0.517	105	0.858	113	0.828
San Martin	31	0.229	55	0.449	119	0.872
Tacna	80	0.591	110	0.899	39	0.286
Tumbes	19	0.140	34	0.278	62	0.454
No Info/Abroad			238		3912	
Total	13542	100	12475	100	17565	100

* Excludes doctors abroad or for whom departmental location is unknown.

TABLE 6.2

Comparison of Census and Sample: Distribution by Sex, Age, Provincial Grouping, and Location vs. Birthplace

	Census		Sample	
	Numbers	Percent	Numbers	Percent
Gender:				
Male	10889	87.287	14705	83.847
Female	1586	12.713	2833	16.153
Total	12475	100	17538	100
Age:				
25-30	2615	21.167	2816	16.261
31-35	2320	18.779	3938	22.741
36-40	1608	13.016	2932	16.931
41-45	1349	10.920	1582	9.136
46-50	1453	11.761	1485	8.575
51-55	1458	11.802	1637	9.453
56-60	780	6.314	1392	8.038
61-65	379	3.068	674	3.892
66+	392	3.173	861	4.972
Total	12354	100	17317	100
Provincial Grouping:				
Lima/Callao	8120	67.008	8616	65.581
Dept. Capitals w/ Med. School	1430	11.801	1697	12.917
Other Department Capitals	1357	11.198	1234	11.334
NonDept. Capitals w/ Hospital	1090	8.995	1234	9.393
NonDept. Capitals w/o Hospital	121	0.999	102	0.776
Total	12118	100	13138	100
Location/Birthplace:				
Currently in Dept. of Birth	5722	47.231	5731	42.065
Currently not in Dept.of Birth	6393	52.769	7893	57.935
Total	12115	100	13624	100

TABLE 6.3

Sub-sectorial Distribution of Doctors

Provincial Grouping	IPSS		MOH		Private	
	Numbers	Percent	Numbers	Percent	Numbers	Percent
Lima/Callao	1230	59.306	2512	69.894	4874	65.221
Dept. Capitals w/ Med. School	259	12.488	307	8.542	1131	15.134
Other Department Capitals	256	12.343	507	14.107	728	9.742
Non-Dept. Capitals w/ Hospital	328	15.815	245	6.817	662	8.859
Non-Dept. Capitals w/o Hospital	1	0.048	23	0.640	78	1.044
Affiliational Totals	2074	100	3594	100	7473	100
Percent of Total	15.8		27.3		56.9	

TABLE 6.4

Location of Doctors by Region *
(in percentages)

Region	IPSS	MOH	Private
Selva	0.1	3.4	4.0
North Sierra	8.4	6.2	3.5
South Sierra	10.1	9.1	9.6
North Coast	13.7	7.0	13.3
Lima Coast	66.0	70.2	66.0
South Coast	1.7	4.0	3.6
Total	100	100	100

* Based on subsample of doctors for whom complete information was available.

TABLE 6.5

Relation of Current Location of Doctors to Place of Birth *
(in percentages)

	IPSS	MOH	Private
In Province of Birth	33.2	34.1	40.1
In Region of Birth but not Province	12.4	9.8	10.2
In Neither Province nor Region	54.4	56.1	49.7
Total	100	100	100

* Based on subsample of doctors for whom complete information was available.

TABLE 6.6

Place of Schooling and Institutional Affiliation of Doctors *
(in percentages)

Place of Study	IPSS	MOH	Private
Lima	66.9	69.9	71.2
Arequipa	6.9	6.4	6.4
Ica	2.9	4.0	3.2
La Libertad	7.3	10.0	8.3
Abroad	15.9	9.6	10.9
Total	100	100	100

* Based on subsample of doctors for whom complete information was available.

TABLE 6.7

Relation Between Current Location and Place of Schooling of Doctors *
(in percentages)

	IPSS	MOH	Private
In Region of Schooling	64.9	62.9	71.5
Not in Region of Schooling	35.1	37.1	28.5
Total	100	100	100

* Based on subsample of doctors for whom complete information was available.

TABLE 6.8

Distribution of Doctors in Relation to Electrification *
(in percentages)

Percent of Homes with Electricity	IPSS Doctors per 10,000 Inhabitants	MOH Doctors per 10,000 Inhabitants	Private Doctors per 10,000 Inhabitants
25% or fewer	0.01	0.19	0.38
Between 25 and 50%	0.18	1.02	1.62
Between 50 and 75%	1.95	1.70	4.28
Greater than 75%	2.61	4.89	9.86
Entire Country	1.24	2.15	4.41

* Based on subsample of doctors for whom complete information was available.

TABLE 6.9

Distribution of Male Doctors by Subsectorial Affiliation
Over Their Working Years

Place of Birth and of Study	Affiliation	Years of Work Experience 0-5	6-10	11-15	16+
Lima	IPSS	2.4	15.7	17.1	61.5
	Ministry	28.8	32.9	31.1	24.7
	Private	68.8	51.4	51.9	61.5
Arequipa	IPSS	07.4	36.8	40.1	34.9
	Ministry	33.6	29.5	27.1	23.2
	Private	59.0	33.7	32.8	41.9

TABLE 6.10

Distribution of Male Doctors by Region Over Their Working Years

Place of Birth
and of Study: Arequipa (South Sierra)

		Years of Work Experience			
Affiliation	Regions	0-5	6-10	11-15	16+
IPSS	Selva	0.8	0.7	0.5	0.3
	N. Sierra	2.1	1.9	1.3	1.0
	S. Sierra	92.8	93.2	95.6	96.3
	N. Coast	2.7	2.5	1.6	1.3
	S. Coast	1.0	0.9	0.6	0.6
	Lima Coast	0.8	0.8	0.5	0.5
Ministry	Selva	3.8	4.0	6.1	6.0
	N. Sierra	4.4	4.5	6.9	6.9
	S. Sierra	71.5	71.3	55.9	55.8
	N. Coast	4.6	4.7	7.2	7.2
	S. Coast	3.8	3.8	5.8	5.8
	Lima Coast	11.9	11.8	18.2	18.3
Private Sector	Selva	3.4	3.1	3.6	3.7
	N. Sierra	4.0	3.8	4.4	4.5
	S. Sierra	78.2	78.7	75.3	75.0
	N. Coast	4.6	4.5	5.2	5.3
	S. Coast	3.4	3.4	3.9	3.9
	Lima Coast	6.4	6.6	7.6	7.5

TABLE 6.11

Distribution of Male Doctors by Province in the South Sierra Over Their Working Years

Place of Birth
and of Study: Arequipa

		Years of Work Experience			
Affiliation	Regions	0-5	6-10	11-15	16+
IPSS	Arequipa	84.8	86.9	93.8	95.5
	Other Department Capitals	10.0	9.6	4.6	4.0
	Other Provinces	5.2	3.5	1.7	0.5
Ministry	Arequipa	97.5	96.3	64.6	68.3
	Other Department Capitals	1.5	1.7	16.4	16.2
	Other Provinces	1.1	2.0	19.1	15.5
Private Sector	Arequipa	87.3	91.7	95.5	94.4
	Other Department Capitals	6.0	5.3	2.8	3.0
	Other Provinces	6.7	3.1	1.7	2.6

TABLE 6.12

Distribution of Male Doctors from Arequipa
with 11-15 Years of Work Experience
by Subsectorial Affiliation and Region

Place of Study: Lima

Affiliation	Percent	Regions	Percent
IPSS	24.1	S. Sierra	79.8
		Lima Coast	6.8
		Other	13.4
Ministry	35.8	S. Sierra	56.2
		Lima Coast	17.9
		Other	25.9
Private Sector	40.1	S. Sierra	48.0
		Lima Coast	26.5
		Other	25.5

TABLE 6.13

Distribution of Male Doctors
with 11-15 Years of Work Experience
and Selected Birthplaces, by Subsectorial Affiliation

	Affiliation		
Place of Birth	IPSS	Ministry	Private
Iquitos	5.8	44.3	49.8
Arequipa	24.1	35.8	40.1
Canas	21.3	37.7	41.0
Lima	17.1	31.1	49.8

TABLE 6.14

Distribution of Male Doctors
with 11-15 Years of Work Experience
with Selected Birthplaces, by Subsectorial Affiliation and Region

Place of Birth	Affiliation	Region of Location		
		S. Sierra	Lima	Other
Arequipa	IPSS	79.8	6.8	13.4
	Ministry	56.2	17.9	25.9
	Private	48.0	26.5	25.5
Canas	IPSS	48.5	17.4	34.1
	Ministry	55.4	18.6	26.0
	Private	36.7	32.3	31.0
Lima	IPSS	9.5	55.7	34.8
	Ministry	8.0	59.5	32.5
	Private	4.2	78.6	17.2

TABLE 6.15

Distribution of Male Doctors
with 11-15 Years Work Experience
from Arequipa or Canas, by Subsectorial Affiliation
and Type of Province

Affiliation	Group of Provinces	Practicing in South Sierra: Place of Birth: Arequipa	Practicing in South Sierra: Place of Birth: Canas	Practicing anywhere in Peru: Place of Birth: Arequipa	Practicing anywhere in Peru: Place of Birth: Canas
IPSS	Capitals	98.4	85.7	78.5	41.6
	Other	1.6	14.3	1.3	6.9
Ministry	Capitals	80.9	60.1	45.5	33.3
	Other	19.1	39.9	22.4	22.1
Private	Capitals	98.3	85.3	47.2	31.3
	Other	1.7	14.7	0.8	5.4

TABLE 6.16

Distribution of Female Doctors from Arequipa with 11-15 Years of Work Experience, Who Studied in Lima, by Subsectorial Affiliation

Affiliation	Percent	Region	Percent
IPSS	0.24	S. Sierra	0.391
		Lima Coast	0.456
		Other	0.153
Ministry	0.413	S. Sierra	0.207
		Lima Coast	0.540
		Other	0.253
Private	0.347	S. Sierra	0.527
		Lima Coast	0.275
		Other	0.198

TABLE 6.17

Distribution of Female Doctors from Arequipa with 11-15 Years of Work Experience, Who Studied in Arequipa, by Subsectorial Affiliation

Affiliation	Percent	Region	Percent
IPSS	0.444	S. Sierra	0.982
		Lima Coast	0.002
		Other	0.016
Ministry	0.286	S. Sierra	0.596
		Lima Coast	0.166
		Other	0.238
Private	0.270	S. Sierra	0.850
		Lima Coast	0.046
		Other	0.104

TABLE 6.18

Distribution of Male Doctors Born and Schooled in Arequipa
and Practicing in the North Coast, by Degree of Electrification of Department

Percentage of Homes with Electricity	Affiliation			Percentage of Regional Population	Ratio of Percentage of Doctors to Percentage of Population		
	IPSS	Ministry	Private		IPSS	Ministry	Private
0 - 25%	1.2	2.4	1.5	45.7	0.026	0.053	0.033
25 - 50%	21.9	43.7	19.9	21.7	1.009	2.014	0.917
50 - 75%	64.2	48.7	64.2	29.8	2.156	1.635	2.154
75 - 100%	12.7	5.2	14.3	2.8	4.607	1.873	5.107

7

The Pharmaceuticals Market

Gary Gereffi

Pharmaceuticals represent between 15 and 20 percent of total health sector expenditures in Peru, a proportion lower than that of most developing countries. The shortage of medicines and other pharmaceutical supplies reflected in this figure is a major constraint to the effective delivery of health services in the country. While about half of the population has access to public sector health care, only about 20 percent of all pharmaceuticals are distributed through governmental programs. For the most part, Peruvians purchase their medicines from private pharmacies. Repeated attempts by the Government of Peru to provide free or low-cost basic medicines to the population through public health and social security programs have been largely unsuccessful. At the same time, the availability of pharmaceuticals in the private sector has also decreased, due to the rising costs of imported materials and governmental price controls on products sold through commercial pharmacies.

This chapter reviews the evolution of low-cost, generic drug programs in Peru within the context of the whole pharmaceuticals market, including the importation and domestic production of pharmaceuticals. First the evolution of essential drugs programs is described. An interesting feature of these programs is that the private sector has generally been called upon to implement them, while in other developing nations government has played a more prominent role in producing and distributing essential drugs (Gereffi 1983a; 1983c; PAHO 1984). For a variety of reasons, the success of Peru's programs has been very limited. The second part of the chapter describes the current structure of and trends in the pharmaceutical industry. Its performance reflects a variety of factors: the size of the domestic market; the relative importance of imports versus domestic production in satisfying national demand for medicines; the roles of the public and private sectors; the prominence of foreign over national manufacturers; the linkages between pharmaceutical suppliers, wholesalers, and retailers; the role of health professionals (especially physicians and pharmacists) in shaping pharmaceutical consumption patterns; and consumer preferences and attitudes toward self-medication and essential drugs. A final section highlights issues affecting the future of the Peruvian pharmaceutical industry.

Growth of the Peruvian Pharmaceutical Industry

As an economic activity, pharmaceutical production is expected to satisfy a country's demand for medicines at reasonable profits to producers and vendors, without placing an undue burden on its balance of payments. From a social perspective, the primary objective is to assure the availability to the population of a sufficient volume of essential medicines, at reasonable cost and of acceptable quality. As governments have attempted to reconcile these economic and social concerns, the pharmaceutical industry—in Peru as in other countries—has found itself in a politically charged environment and subject to a high degree of government scrutiny and control. The availability of pharmaceuticals in Peru can be understood only by looking at the ongoing interplay of these divergent objectives and interests.

Pharmaceutical production in Peru began in the late 1940s, and by 1960, several pharmaceutical plants supplied about 15 percent of the total amount of medicines consumed nationally. More rapid growth followed; between 1960 and 1970, the output of pharmaceutical firms increased at an annual rate of nearly 17 percent, more than double the 8 percent annual growth rate for the manufacturing sector as a whole. Pharmaceutical production also exceeded the chemical industry's 12.5 percent annual rate of growth (Vega-Centeno and Remenyi 1980: 35-36). But this expansion slowed after 1970 as the result of a law that relegated the pharmaceuticals industry to a secondary level of economic priority, thus making it ineligible for a number of investment and tax incentives it had previously enjoyed. At the same time, new restrictions regulating the activities of subsidiaries of transnational corporations in Peru were issued. Since many of the pharmaceutical firms in the country were foreign-owned, these measures tended to limit the industry's expansion.

During the 1960s and early 1970s, raw materials and packaging accounted for about 45 percent of the total production costs in the industry. Over 90 percent of the raw materials (*i.e.*, active and inert ingredients) used in pharmaceutical manufacture were imported, but between 75 and 80 percent of the packaging materials were produced locally (Vega-Centeno and Remenyi 1980:43-45). From 1976 to 1983, raw materials alone accounted for between 45 and 60 percent of pharmaceutical production costs, packaging materials for 11-15 percent, labor costs for 6-9 percent, and general administrative expenditures on the order of 11-14 percent (Price Waterhouse 1984). An additional production cost factor was the foreign exchange cost incurred on imported items due to the continuous devaluation of the Peruvian currency during this period; the magnitude of this factor fluctuated between 7 and 23 percent of overall production costs (1). The imported share of the raw materials utilized in the pharmaceutical industry was between 90 and 94 percent.

When one considers that imported inputs are primarily active ingredients without which Peru's pharmaceutical industry could not function, the true nature of the country's import dependency becomes apparent. To date only a few firms have been able or willing to manufacture active ingredients in Peru. The result has been a deteriorating balance of payments position for the industry, as it continues to generate large deficits in the absence of substantial import substituting or exporting efforts.

A problem related to this import dependency concerns price controls. With one-half to two-thirds of the pharmaceutical industry's production costs determined directly or indirectly by imported materials, and with devaluations of the Peruvian currency at average rates of well over 100 percent annually for the past several years, it is obvious that pharmaceutical manufacturers have had to press for continuous price escalations for many of the medicines sold within Peru (particularly the ethical or prescription pharmaceuticals, which tend to be the most import-intensive). At the same time, however, the government has been under great pressure to keep pharmaceutical prices down, since spiraling inflation has continued to erode Peruvians' purchasing power. Between 1980 and 1984, the cumulative rate of inflation in Peru was about 2,200 percent (*Informe de Gerencia* 1985:4). Industry and government are thus in conflict as each responds to pressures that move them in opposing directions.

The erosion of purchasing power caused by inflation, especially since 1980 (2), has adversely affected direct health care expenditures more than other items in the household budget. In 1984, health care expenditures by urban households accounted for just 2.6 percent of total household expenditures, and pharmaceuticals accounted for one-half of this proportion, or 1.3 percent (ENNSA 1984). This average for health care expenditures as a proportion of all household spending is three-fourths of the national average in 1972 (2.6 vs. 3.45 percent), and is even less than the average spent by the poorest decile of the population in 1972 (2.9 percent) (ENCA 1972).

Generic Drugs in the Public Sector

In 1985, President Alan Garcia named as his new Minister of Health the internationally respected former Deputy Director of the World Health Organization, Dr. David Tejada de Rivero. A major supporter of WHO's Action Program on Essential Drugs, Dr. Tejada stated that one of his key objectives as minister would be to assure that "there will be an adequate supply of medicines corresponding to the real and most pressing needs of the national majority, that these medicines will reach the remotest corners of the country for those that need them, and that these medicines will be economically accessible to the people" (Guerrero 1985). Like his predecessors over the past quarter-century, Dr. Tejada believes that an adequate supply of pharmaceuticals—the right drugs, at the right time, in the right place, and at the right price—is critical to improving Peru's desperate health situation. What needs to be determined is why the essential drugs programs have failed to work in the past, despite major commitments in this area by previous governments.

Social Medicines

Peru's experience with essential medicines has its origins in a 1959 law (*Ley* 13200), authorizing the Ministry of Health (MOH) to classify a set of pharmaceutical items as essential for the recovery of health. In 1960, the MOH selected 20 "social" medicines, to be produced by private firms and delivered, every three months, to health posts in low-income areas and to government-owned hospitals at no more than a third the price of comparable brand-name drugs. In 1962, this collaboration between the MOH and the private sector was formalized (*Decreto Supremo* 566) as the Social Medicines Program. It included 53 products and 69 dosage form pharmaceuticals (primarily symptomatic medicines and some antibiotics), whose sale price to the public was not to exceed 50 percent of the price of similar brand-name products. In 1969, the program was extended once more (*Decreto Supremo* 00160-69); the MOH was authorized to convoke public tenders for the supply of pharmaceuticals, with the distribution outlets to include retail pharmacies and *boticas* (3).

But the Social Medicines Program never attained acceptance by health professionals or the population in general. Since the program was voluntary and poorly coordinated, the supply of these drugs was erratic and insufficient. The distribution channels did not allow for full coverage of the target population, and there was a recurrent shortage of operating funds since many of the drugs were dispensed *gratis* or at very low prices. In addition, the products included in the program were criticized for not addressing the primary therapeutic needs of the population.

Basic Medicines

Evolution during the 1970s. The notion of low-priced medicines for the economically disadvantaged was retained as a high priority by the military government that assumed power in 1968. Its Global Development Plan for 1971-1975 provided the context for a new Basic Medicines Program, created in 1971 and structured quite differently from its predecessors. During its first phase, between 1971 and 1975, this program was established as an independent entity managed directly by the military government. In order to guide the selection and acquisition process, an official list (*petitorio*) of "basic" medicines, including 185 pharmaceutical products available in 265 different dosage forms, was drawn up in 1971 by a specially-appointed commission of medical experts. In 1975, the Basic Medicines Program was placed under the jurisdiction of the reinstituted MOH Pharmacy Division (*Decreto Supremo* 0045-75), which had been disbanded between 1968-1975. The MOH was thus given full administrative, financial, and operative control over all aspects of the program.

The main mechanism for the provision of "basic" medicines was a series of public tenders open to drug companies located in Peru. These public tenders varied in their timing and duration as well as in the number of products covered by each (Table 7.1). There was a tendency for the number of items included to increase during the first five years of the program, although the number of "basic" medicines actually bid upon by participating firms was always less than the total listed in the *petitorio*—itself growing in size and changing in composition each year.

It is difficult, on the basis of Table 7.1, to determine trends in terms of the value and volume of "basic" medicines covered by the public tenders. The value of the bids for supplying these products increased greatly in current *soles* between 1971-1980, but if these amounts are converted into constant *soles* to control for inflation, the total value of the tenders appears to decline. Expressed in terms of US dollars, there was a drop in value from $35.5 million in 1975-1976 to $27.6 million in 1978-1979. The best measure of the growth or decline in "basic" medicines would be the number of units encompassed by the bids, but those data are unavailable.

The users of "basic" medicines were primarily public sector institutions, with additional sales through a few selected pharmacies and *boticas* in Lima, Ica, and Ancash. Table 7.2 shows that within the public sector the Peruvian Social Security Institute (IPSS) accounted for 56 percent of the sales of "basic" medicines between 1979 and 1983, the MOH for 36 percent, the Armed Forces and Police for 4 percent, and other public institutions for the remaining 4 percent. In constant *soles* however, the volume of sales continued to decline; by 1981, sales were only two-thirds as great in real terms as they had been in 1979; and by 1983, when the program was phased out, "basic" medicines sales in constant *soles* were only one-third of their value four years earlier.

The participation of Peruvian drug companies in the 1978-1979 public tender (Table 7.3) was slightly greater than that of the foreign pharmaceutical subsidiaries established in the country. However, a considerable proportion of actual pharmaceutical production in Peru is carried out for foreign firms on a subcontracting basis by local companies. Thus the importance of Peruvian firms (*e.g.*, their proportion of Efesa, Farmindustria, Magma, Lusa, and Sanitas) in terms of *value added* is far greater than final sales of "basic" medicines might indicate (Vega-Centeno and Remenyi 1980:48-49) (4).

Political Discontinuities. In order to understand why the impact of the Basic Medicines Program was limited from its 1971 inception, and why the program waned in the final years before its dismantling in the early 1980s, we must take into account a wide variety of economic, technical, political, and cultural factors that individually and jointly affect the selection, acquisition, distribution, and use of "basic" medicines. At the most general level, Peru's efforts to provide essential medicines to its populace have been marked by sharp political discontinuities. This is true not only *between* programs ("social," "basic," or "essential" medicines), but also *within* each of these programs. During the military governments of 1968-1980, there were seven different Ministers of Health, making the establishment of a coordinated "basic" medicines policy difficult. The key transition point for the program, however, came in 1975, when it was incorporated into the MOH's Pharmacy Division.

This change was significant for two reasons. First, the government now seemed to adopt a more accommodating attitude toward the interests of private pharmaceutical firms regarding their participation in the Basic Medicines Program. Ultimately, this increasingly cooperative relationship ran aground on the issue of price controls in the industry (to be discussed in detail in the following section). However, it is significant that private companies felt the system of public tenders was improved in the late 1970s in some important respects. Manufacturers, for example, were allowed to use their corporate and product brand names on the packages and labels for "basic" medicines; previously, only information directly related to the generic product had been permitted. In addition, a system of regular price adjustments was established for pharmaceutical producers who were largely dependent on imported raw materials. This was a step forward in principle, as the manufacturers saw it, although the actual implementation of these price increases did not proceed smoothly in practice.

The second important result of the 1975 transition was that the direction of the Basic Medicines Program was centered in the MOH. While this opened up the possibility that the public sector pharmaceutical supply could be better coordinated with other elements of the government's health policy, it also led to conflicts involving the pharmaceutical industry (for example, over price controls), other public sector institutions (such as the IPSS and eventually the Ministry of Industry), health professionals (especially physicians), and consumers of "basic" medicines, over issues such as quality control and the adequate supply and distribution of these products.

The problems in the functioning of this program were not the fault of any one group. Whereas the Social Medicines Program of the 1960s relied on the voluntary participation of some private companies to supply drugs to a relatively small group of indigent clients served mainly by the MOH, the Basic Medicines Program called for a more formal participation of the industry to answer the needs of all public sector institutions, including IPSS, the Armed Forces, and the Police. Some private sector producers complained that this broadened program cut too deeply into their commercial market for medicines, since most members of the Armed Forces and Police were by no means indigent and could afford to purchase brand-name drugs. However, estimates of the share of "basic" medicines in relation to the total output of the pharmaceutical industry during this period are below 10 percent of total sales (Garrido-Lecca 1984:36).

Economic Problems. A fundamental problem in structuring the public tenders was that information on the consumption of pharmaceuticals by various public sector institutions was practically non-existent in the beginning of the 1970s. Even today, reliable consumption figures are difficult to obtain. It is only in the past few years that the MOH and IPSS have been able to centralize requests for drugs by regional hospitals and health centers on a periodic basis; prior to this, each unit submitted its own orders for the products it felt it needed, thus eliminating the possibility of savings from bulk purchasing. Because these public institutions generally did not have enough money to buy more than a fraction of the drugs they required, we have no way of knowing what their *real* demand for pharmaceuticals was. When drug supplies did arrive, they were quickly exhausted, usually by the largest institutions in major urban areas. Rarely did "basic" medicines reach the rural population.

When the Basic Medicines Program was established, it was granted no working capital by the government, nor did it have an initial stock of pharmaceuticals from which to supply its clients on a replacement basis. Eventually, a minimal amount of working capital was obtained via a ministerial resolution requiring all public health institutions to turn over to the program two-thirds of their budgets for a year for laboratory supplies and radio- graphic materials. Subsequently, the program was supposed to derive its operating budget from consumers, who would pay a small amount over the price at which the manufacturers agreed to supply "basic" medicines to the program (PAHO 1975:21,13-14). But since most of the program's clients were unable to pay anything for the medicines they received, this method of funding was inadequate, and the program was generally underfinanced as a result.

The price of "basic" medicines was considerably less than similar brand-name drugs, with average savings of about 35 percent (PAHO 1975:17), due both to the reduced profit margins accepted by private pharmaceutical companies and to the almost total absence of marketing expenditures for the program (for samples, medical representatives, advertising, fancy labels or containers, etc.). Many in the industry felt that this inattention to elementary marketing principles reinforced the idea in the minds of even poor consumers that "basic" medicines were inferior because they were cheap. In addition, Peru's reliance on imported inputs meant that pharmaceutical prices were generally being pushed upward, and this too contributed to a lessening of the appeal of "basic" medicines, since the purchasing power of the population continued to decline and the pharmaceutical industry was increasingly reluctant to participate in the face of rising input costs while final product prices were being controlled.

Essential Medicines

When the Belaunde government took office in 1980, it inherited the Basic Medicines Program from the military era—just as the first "social" medicines program had remained in effect for a few years after the military assumed power in 1968. The Basic Medicines Program was running into a number of difficulties by 1980, however, particularly with respect to price controls. Because "basic" (and later "essential") medicines were sold to the government at prices below those of similar brand-name drugs on the market, price controls on brand-name pharmaceuticals in effect froze the price of the generic medicines at levels that manufacturers insisted were below their production costs. This factor, together with a backlog of late payments and the consequent erosion of credit to public sector clients, led drug companies to withdraw gradually from the Basic Medicines program, which came to a virtual halt by 1982.

The legal and administrative groundwork for a new Essential Medicines Program was established in June, 1982. The objective of the program was to assure a permanent supply of essential drugs at reasonable prices for the entire population, with an emphasis on the primary levels of health care. Like the Basic Medicines Program, the supply of "essential" medicines was to come mainly from private drug companies, which would submit bids through a public tender system. Unlike the previous program, however, these were to be *international* public tenders open to any drug company in the world (as opposed to the *national* public tenders of the Basic Medicines Program, which excluded the participation of firms not physically located in Peru). The major advantage of this scheme, supposedly, was that it would mean the lowest possible prices to the government. (Dr. Uriel Garcia, Minister of Health from 1980-1982, published several articles in *Caretas* showing average price differentials of 200 percent between "basic" medicines and generic drugs offered by WHO. Aspirin, for example, was seven times more expensive when produced in Peru than it would have been if it were imported.)

However, there were drawbacks to the new program. One was that the international bids had to be made in *soles*. Given the instability of the *sol* at the time, most foreign manufacturers were reluctant to participate in the bidding on this basis. The scheme also encountered resistance because it provided a disincentive for the creation of local manufacturing capacity. Peruvian companies were especially concerned because they had no other option but to produce for the local market.

The first public tender under the Essential Medicines Program took place in June, 1983. It was supposedly international, but no foreign companies presented bids. The 39 domestic drug firms that initially participated submitted acceptable bids on only 31 of the 246 products open to tender offers; direct negotiations with companies produced contracts for another 140 "essential" medicines, bringing the total number of products adjudicated in this first tender to 171 (Gálvez de Llaque and Fefer 1985:2). The official list of "essential" medicines included 253 generic products in 368 dosage forms, thus making it considerably larger than the initial *petitorio* for "basic" medicines.

The quarterly sales of "essential" medicines in Peru in 1984 are shown in Table 7.4. The total sales for the year, 1,739.2 million (constant 1980) *soles*, equals approximately US $6 million. Since all pharmaceutical sales in Peru in 1984 equaled US $200 million (private and public sectors), "essential" medicines represented about 3 percent of the pharmaceutical market—a low proportion compared to the 6-9 percent overall market share of "basic" medicines in the 1970s. Nearly half (48 percent) of all essential medicines went to the IPSS, 37 percent to the MOH, and 9 and 6 percent, respectively, to the Armed Forces and Police. This is similar to the institutional breakdown for "basic" medicines (Table 7.2), except that IPSS received relatively fewer "essential" medicines and the Armed Forces and Police proportionately more.

The extent of participation of local and foreign pharmaceutical companies in the Essential Medicines Program is shown in Table 7.5. Locally-owned firms accounted for two-thirds of the contracts awarded in 1983, with foreign firms established in Peru gaining contracts amounting to about one-third of the total. The role of local private companies thus appears somewhat greater in the Essential Medicines Program than it was under the Basic Medicines Program (see Table 7.3).

Like its predecessors, the Essential Medicines Program never lived up to the expectations—whether measured in terms of volume of overall sales, extent of participation by private companies, coverage of the rural and urban-marginal population, acceptance by health professionals and consumers, or degree of coordination among public sector health institutions—of those who created it, and the program was terminated by the Garcia administration in 1985, just two years after its inception. Why, given its need for large quantities of reliable, low-cost generic medicines, has Peru been unable to structure and implement a workable essential drugs program? The following factors are relevant in providing an answer to this question.

Effects of Price Controls. With the exception of two medium-sized, state-owned laboratories, Lusa (Laboratorios Unidos, S. A.) and Indumil (Industrias Militares), the public sector in Peru has no pharmaceuticals production capability. Nor does the state have a system in place for the distribution of medicines. Instead, the government, through its Essential Medicines Program, sponsors the procurement from private manufacturers of finished products that can be distributed to public sector institutions.

The fact that in Peru cooperation with the private sector is required for the production and distribution of essential medicines makes such programs vulnerable to factors perceived as creating a negative investment climate for the country's pharmaceutical industry. In this regard, government price controls have clearly had a pernicious effect on the availability of "essential" medicines. There was a period between 1982 and 1984 when the effective control over pharmaceutical prices was lodged in two ministries: the Ministry of Industry (for locally-produced drugs and inputs) and the MOH (for finished, imported pharmaceuticals). This created considerable confusion, exacerbated by mixed signals about the magnitude of, and delays in the timing of, price increases.

In 1984, when price controls were again consolidated in the MOH, a polynomial formula was devised to guide price increases for medicines (5). According to this formula, the allowable monthly price increase was based on the assumption that imported inputs account for about 40 percent of average drug production costs. The formula was to be applied automatically every 30 days to all ethical drugs. In fact, however, it was applied only sporadically, so that the prices of many brand-name products on the market remained frozen for as long as 18 months.

The slowness of the government in granting price increases had several negative effects. When price increases were finally granted, the accumulated readjustment rate often led to new prices that appeared excessively high, thus exposing companies receiving increases to hostile criticism and charges of exploitation. The response by a number of firms was to stop or slow down local sales of the drugs whose prices were frozen, and sometimes to introduce new but similar products into the market that would be free of controls and thus could be sold at higher prices. This led at times to a shortage of some of the best-selling pharmaceuticals in Peru.

Although "essential" medicines were supposed to be *price regulators* for brand-name drugs, they produced the opposite effect, as the artificially low prices for brand-name items restricted the availability of generic substitutes. Some "essential" medicines could not be sold because their prices, which by law could not exceed those of the most economical brand-name equivalents on the market, had already risen (at the maximum allowed rate of up to 4 percent per month) to a point at which essential drugs were more expensive than some of their brand-name equivalents. In 1985, 31 of 171 "essential" medicines could not be sold in Peru because their official prices were *higher* than those of their brand-name equivalents (Gálvez de Llaque and Fefer 1985:5). Obviously, if a significant price differential cannot be maintained between generic and brand-name items, the single most important benefit of "essential" medicines—low price—ceases to exist.

Resistance from Health Professionals. Another problem encountered by the Essential Medicines Program, like its forerunners, was that it faced considerable resistance from health professionals. Most physicians dislike restrictions placed on their discretionary ability to prescribe the products they deem appropriate for their patients. A complaint about essential drugs programs in general is that they limit the selection of medicines used by public sector institutions to official drug lists that contain only generic items, thus making it impossible for participating physicians to prescribe some of the most popular brand-name drugs available on the market. One observer of the current scene in Peru feels that the MOH generated additional resentment among physicians because it failed to consult the Peruvian Medical Association (*Colegio Médico*) when designing the Essential Medicines Program (Garrido-Lecca 1984:45-46).

The Medical Association's perception of having been ignored reflects a long-standing professional rivalry between physicians and pharmacists over the direction of Peru's essential drugs programs. Since 1975, when the Basic Medicines Program was placed under the control of the Pharmacy Division in the MOH, pharmacists have taken the lead in running government programs supplying generic pharmaceuticals to public sector institutions. Pharmacists who do not work for the government, however, do not have such a uniformly favorable attitude toward the essential drugs programs. The reason is that many pharmacists own drugstores, and since 1975 drugstores have had to charge a 25 percent markup on all retail sales of pharmaceuticals (*Resolución Suprema* 104-75). Since the income of drugstore owners is a direct percentage of total sales, the prevailing incentive structure favors the sale of higher-priced over lower-priced medicines (in contrast, for example, to a system in which pharmacists earn a fixed amount for every prescription filled, regardless of price). If generic medicines are ever to gain widespread popularity and acceptance in Peru, the incentive structure for pharmacists at the retail level will probably have to be changed.

Consumer Attitudes. Another factor leading to a low level of acceptance of essential drugs in Peru is the attitude of consumers themselves, who believe (in part perhaps because of what some physicians and pharmacists tell them) that generics are inferior because they are cheap. In fact, there have been some well-publicized problems in the quality control of "basic" as well as "essential" medicines. Nonetheless, the overall quality of Peru's essential drugs appears acceptable, especially when the suppliers are large, established pharmaceutical companies who do much of their own quality control. A number of prominent suppliers have certified that they use exactly the same inputs and production processes in making essential drugs as they do in producing their brand-name items; only the packaging and the price differ.

The biggest problem with the low level of acceptance of essential drugs among consumers may not be quality so much as image. There has been almost no attention given in these programs to marketing the products in an effective and appealing way. It is tempting to think that because public sector institutions constitute a "captive market" for essential drugs, no promotion of these programs or their products is necessary, but this is not the case. There is considerable evidence that even very poor consumers exercise the option of buying more expensive brand-name pharmaceuticals when they feel that lower-priced products are not as good. There have been proposals from some of Peru's private pharmaceutical firms to promote essential drugs programs to the general public at relatively low cost, but so far none of these has been accepted by the MOH. The cooperation of local suppliers and affiliated health professionals will be needed if the image of essential drugs programs in Peru is to take a positive turn.

Lack of Coordination. A final reason for Peru's limited success in implementing essential drugs programs is the lack of coordination among public sector institutions. The conflict between the MOH and the Ministry of Industry over the administration of price controls has already been mentioned, and there are equally serious conflicts within the health sector itself. The MOH and IPSS, for instance, have perennially been at odds over policy matters. The Ministry is responsible for national health sector policy, yet its economic resources are in no way commensurate with its responsibilities. The IPSS budget for medical care in general, and medicines in particular, is greater than that of the MOH (see Tables 7.6 and 7.7), despite the fact that social security in Peru covers only about 18 percent of the population while the MOH is responsible for providing health services for at least 50 percent (6). IPSS, the Armed Forces, and the Police have guarded their substantial political and economic autonomy. To take but one example, each of these three public institutions has its own official drug list to guide its procurement of generic and brand-name medicines; there is still no unified *petitorio* for the public sector, which of course undercuts the impact of the essential drugs programs.

The Peruvian Pharmaceutical Industry

Market Size and Structure

The structure of the pharmaceutical industry in Peru is quite similar to that of other Latin American countries (see Table 7.6), although the total number of Peruvian firms is comparatively small. In most Latin American countries, private sector sales far exceed public (including social security medical care programs). Peru's market concentration is not very strong, in that the largest 20-25 producers account for only about two-thirds of total sales. The market share of wholly-owned domestic firms is relatively small at around 25 percent, leaving the industry exposed to foreign control (7).

Although precise figures are hard to come by, only about 10 percent of finished pharmaceutical products consumed in Peru are imported, while 90 percent of products sold undergo some degree of local manufacture, usually involving relatively simple formulation and packaging activities. The situation is quite different, though, if one focuses on pharmaceutical inputs rather than finished drugs. Raw material costs account for about half of total production costs. The share of these inputs produced in Peru is minimal, fluctuating from 6-10 percent in recent years. Most pharmaceutical inputs used in the country are imported.

Among the several government institutions involved, IPSS accounts for about 70 percent of the total public sector demand for drugs. MOH hospitals and health centers represent about 20 percent of the demand for medicines by government institutions, and the Armed Forces and other public agencies account for the remaining 10 percent. This contrasts sharply with the respective population coverage of the MOH and IPSS: 27 and 18 percent, respectively.

Pharmaceutical Sales Trends, 1977-1984

A general summary of sales trends in Peru's pharmaceutical market between 1977 and 1984 is provided in Table 7.7. It should be noted that these data refer only to private pharmacy sales (about 72 percent of all pharmaceutical sales in Peru); the total size of the market is approximately one-third larger than these figures indicate. Private pharmacy sales in Peru stood at just under US $145 million in 1984. Ethical pharmaceutical products represent 94 percent of this amount ($135.2 million), and over-the-counter (OTC) products six percent ($9.1 million). Of 105 million units sold in 1984, 92 million (87 percent) were ethical pharmaceuticals and 13 million (13 percent) were OTC products.

Total pharmacy sales in Peru increased 14 percent from 1977 (US $126.1 million) to 1984 (U.S.$144.4 million). However, the number of units sold decreased by 22 percent during these same years, from 134.3 million units in 1977 to 105.3 million units in 1984. These same trends are reflected in the ethical as well as the OTC markets. The dramatic rise in the value of pharmacy sales in current *soles* during this period is due to the very high rates of inflation in Peru after 1978.

Pharmaceutical sales reached a peak in 1980. From then on there has been a steady decline in the value as well as the volume of sales. The value of pharmacy sales dropped 18 percent from 1980 ($175.8 million) to 1984 ($144.4 million), while the volume of sales fell even more sharply, registering a 37 percent decline (from 168.3 million units in 1980 to 105.3 million units in 1984). Table 7.8 shows that this market contraction, while generally severe, has been even more detrimental to the output of OTC products than ethical pharmaceuticals; the average decrease in the volume of medicines sold since 1980 was 37 percent, but the sales decline was 34 percent for ethical pharmaceuticals and 55 percent for OTC products. This is particularly significant for the lower income groups in Peru, because the average unit price of OTC items is between one-third and one-half that of ethical pharmaceuticals (Gereffi 1983d, Table 2.2).

The average unit price of pharmaceuticals as a whole rose substantially between 1979-1981, and again in 1984, which contributed to a decrease in *per capita* pharmaceutical consumption during the 1980-1984 period (see Table 7.9). In US dollars, the decline was from $10.16 in 1980 to $7.52 in 1984 (26 percent), while in units the drop was even more severe, from 9.7 to 5.5 (44 percent). The increase in the unit price of pharmaceuticals in Peru is explained in large part by persistent inflation coupled with devaluation (which has a particularly strong impact on the pharmaceutical industry because of its high degree of dependence on imported inputs), and by the elevated cost of commercial credit needed to finance the imports.

Table 7.10 compares the increase in pharmaceutical prices from 1976 to 1983 with changes in the cost-of-living index and the exchange rate in Peru. The index for pharmaceutical prices during this period rose from 100 to 2,206, but the cost-of-living and exchange rate indices climbed even more sharply. The cost-of-living index increased more than thirty-five-fold between 1976 and 1983, while Peru's currency was devalued by a factor of almost 30 during the same seven-year period. In almost every year, pharmaceutical prices rose less rapidly than the prices of other goods and services represented in the cost-of-living index.

The rise and subsequent decline in Peru's pharmaceutical market during the 1977-1984 period reflects a combination of factors. First, the economy briefly appeared to be on the upswing in 1979 and 1980, due in part to favorable commodity prices and external loan agreements. In addition, 1980 marked the return of democratic government; the Belaunde administration took office in July, and municipal elections were held the following November. Due to electoral pressures, substantial price increases for a number of products, including drugs, were delayed until 1981, but in May and October of that year pharmaceutical price increases of 18 percent and 21 percent, respectively, were authorized by the government. This helps to explain the relatively sharp decline in the volume of units sold in 1981, while the value of pharmaceutical sales in US dollars remained relatively high. From 1982 to 1984, both the value and volume of pharmaceutical sales continued to drop (8).

Some of the foreign-owned laboratories, in apparent response to the contraction of the Peruvian pharmaceuticals market, have discontinued their operations in the country and have sold their manufacturing plants to local private companies. Recent examples of this include the transfer of Cyanamid Peruana's production installations to Quimica Suiza, and the sale of Merck, Sharp & Dohme's plant to Medifarma.

The Major Pharmaceutical Suppliers

There are approximately 155 pharmaceutical companies registered in Peru, of which about 70 actually formulate pharmaceutical products for human use. Those with manufacturing plants in Peru either formulate their own product lines or engage in contract manufacturing for laboratories without production facilities. Companies manufacturing and marketing their own product lines include Roussel, Hoechst, Schering A.G., Ciba-Geigy, Squibb, Parke Davis, Farmindustria, and Abeefe; companies that manufacture extensively for third parties include Alfa, Efesa, Farmitalia, and Pfizer. Among the laboratories that do not make their own pharmaceuticals locally but have a strong sales representation in Peru are Eli Lilly, Upjohn, Schering, Cyanamid, Imperial Chemical Industries, Glaxo, and Boehringer Ingelheim.

Table 7.11 identifies the major pharmaceutical companies in Peru by nationality, and identifies those that have manufacturing operations in the country. American and European subsidiaries of large transnational drug firms predominate, especially in the ethical pharmaceuticals sector (9). Nationally-owned companies, even though they represent 50 percent of total investments in the industry, account for about 40 percent of the volume and only 15 percent of the value of drug sales (Gereffi 1983d:2.15). It is interesting to note that all of the major Peruvian drug firms have their own production plants, and many engage in third-party manufacturing for transnational laboratories.

Wholesale Distributors and Pharmacies

There are five major wholesale distributors of pharmaceutical products in Peru: Quimica Suiza, Grupo Ferreyros, Richard O. Custer, Drogueria Kahan, and Albis S.A. All are Peruvian owned, although Quimica Suiza and Albis are reported to be joint ventures with Swiss investors. Quimica Suiza, Grupo Ferreyros, Richard O. Custer, and Drogueria Kahan are highly diversified companies. Besides supplying pharmaceuticals, they deal in a wide range of other product lines: cosmetics, liquor, dry goods, veterinary products, agrochemicals, kitchen appliances, heavy equipment, etc. The only distributor that has specialized entirely in pharmaceuticals for human use is Albis.

The most decentralized of the distributors is Grupo Ferreyros, also known as Efesa (Enrique Ferreyros S.A.). It is made up of six distributors serving different regions of the country: Norfesa, Surfesa, Centrofesa, Codina, Ferreyco, and Difesa. Overall, Efesa utilizes a network of 13 warehouses spread across the country. Grupo Ferreyros also includes a laboratory that does considerable contract manufacturing of pharmaceutical products for companies without their own industrial plants in Peru. Quimica Suiza, which is the largest of the national distributors, appears to have a very centralized structure. The most diversified of the wholesalers, it is reported also to have acquired some manufacturing capability. Richard O. Custer distributes 4,000 items and deals with nearly 50 local drug firms.

The trend toward developing integrated manufacturing and wholesaler operations is most pronounced in the two largest nationally-owned pharmaceutical companies, Farmindustria and Abeefe. Both are family firms. Farmindustria was founded in 1956 by the family that set up Drogueria Kahan five years earlier, primarily as a distributor of OTC products. Today 55 percent of Drogueria Kahan's sales come from Farmindustria production, 30 percent from products made by other local pharmaceutical companies, and 15 percent from finished drugs directly imported from abroad. Abeefe's pharmaceutical output is channeled through its own wholesale distributor, Perufarma.

Pharmacies generally depend on the extension of credit from wholesalers, typically for 15 days; public sector institutions may receive credit for up to 30 days. There are no major pharmacy chains in Peru as there are in other LAC countries (such as Mexico). By law, only licensed pharmacists can open a pharmacy (see Bates 1983). An interesting topic worthy of further investigation is the extent to which savings could be achieved through economies of scale at the retail outlet level if existing pharmacies were to affiliate in larger groupings that would permit the pooled purchasing of drugs. One reason why this may not occur is that the standard 25 percent mark-up allowed to pharmacies rewards the dispenser for selling higher-priced medicines. If more sales of lower-priced drugs are to be encouraged, a careful analysis of the pricing mechanism at the retail level is needed.

Summary and Conclusions

The pharmaceutical industry in Peru is divided into two distinct segments: the private sector market, which accounts for about three-quarters of overall drug sales, and the public sector market, accounting for slightly less than a quarter of sales. Although the number of drug companies operating in the country is sizeable, the market is relatively small in international terms. In addition, sales trends in the industry have been sharply downward between 1980 and 1984, primarily reflecting the economic recession and consequent decrease in purchasing power of the population. Many firms have cut back their operations, and a few have withdrawn from the market altogether. A major problem, from the companies' point of view, is governmental price regulation, which has been administered somewhat erratically. An improvement in the price control area, beginning with a *regular schedule* of permissible increases if the controls are to be retained, would go a long way toward facilitating a better understanding and working relationship between the industry and the government.

The public sector market, although accounting for only a quarter of national sales, has been the object of a series of initiatives by the government to establish an effective essential drugs program. These efforts have met with relatively little success. Although a large proportion of both foreign and locally-owned drug firms operating in the country have participated in these schemes, local private companies have a particularly strong interest in cooperating with the government to make these programs work, since public sector institutions represent a larger share of their total sales than they do for foreign companies.

Here again, price controls emerge as a problem. Because the price increases on ethical products have not been authorized on a regular basis (in effect, freezing the price of ethical drugs for extended periods of time), a number of "essential" medicines have *higher* prices than their brand-name equivalents, thus preventing the "essential" medicines from being sold in the market. The private companies, both local and foreign, have offered on various occasions to cooperate with the government to establish an effective essential drugs program *if* certain conditions are met. One is the removal or reduction of price controls on their ethical medicines, in return for supporting a program offering essential drugs to the public sector. In addition, the private companies would like to see an essential medicines program limited to the economically most needy groups in the country. More specifically, they appear to support such a program for MOH hospitals and clinics, but they resist extending low-priced essential drugs to IPSS, the Armed Forces, and the Police, which the drug companies claim can afford commercially priced medicines.

The many problems that have plagued Peru's essential drugs efforts are rooted in the relationship between the government and the pharmaceutical industry, in the role that health professionals (physicians and pharmacists) play in these programs, in the largely negative attitudes of consumers toward essential drugs, and in conflicts between public sector institutions. Most of these problems are resolvable if greater collaboration among the involved parties can be attained.

One option that apparently has not been pursued in Peru is the development of a broad-based program of generic medicines, which could be sold in both the public and the private sectors. The generic drugs industry has been growing very rapidly in a number of industrialized countries, with considerable economic benefits for consumers. The capability of producing generics is already present in Peru, and this would seem to be a useful alternative to explore to make pharmaceutical products available at competitive prices to all segments of the Peruvian population.

Footnotes

1. The following gives a sense of the evolution of pharmaceutical production costs during this period:

	1976 (Constant 1983 *Soles*)	%	1983 (Constant 1983 *Soles*)	%
Raw Materials	40,071	52	46,673	45
Exchange Rate Costs	7,997	10	23,709	23
Subtotal	48,068	62	70,382	68
Packaging Materials	11,647	15	11,965	11
Labor	7,119	9	8,505	8
General Expenditures	11,221	14	13,666	13
Total	78,055	100	104,518	100

(Source: Price Waterhouse 1984: Table 4.1)

2. The inflation rate in 1985 was approximately 160 percent, an increase of 43 percent over the 1984 rate of 111.5 percent.

3. There are three kinds of retail sales outlets for drugs in Peru. *Pharmacies* are establishments owned by pharmacists and theoretically staffed by them, which sell the whole range of ethical and over-the-counter products. *Boticas* may be owned by anyone, but are supposed to be staffed by pharmacists; they sell the same range of products as pharmacies. *Botiquines* are located in a variety of institutional settings (from factories to rural health facilities), are staffed by pharmaceutical auxiliaries, and sell a restricted range of products. For a recent analysis of Peruvian pharmacies, see Bates 1983.

4. The legal guidelines for the public tenders on "basic" medicines prohibited the subcontracting of winning bids by pharmaceutical manufacturers, but this rule apparently was often ignored.

5. The formula is as follows:

$$P_t = P_o\,(0.4\,d + 0.6\,i) \times \frac{0.9}{100}$$

where:

P_t = Readjusted price
P_o = Price before the readjustment
d = Percentage of devaluation of the *sol* vis-a-vis the U.S. dollar, at the official exchange rate
i = Percentage of inflation, based on the Consumer Price Index of Metropolitan Lima

The devaluation and inflation indices should correspond to the month prior to the application for the readjustment.

6. Actual coverage is only 27 percent.

7. For other international comparisons, see Gereffi 1983b, 1985.

8. Preliminary data from 1985 point to a possible reversal of this downward trend.

9. For evidence of a similar pattern of American and European leadership in the pharmaceutical industry at the global level, see Gereffi 1982.

TABLE 7.1

Public Tenders for Basic Medicines in Peru, 1971–1980
(Millions of Current Soles)

Public tenders	Amount	Increase	Total	Number of Pharma-ceutical products	Number of dosage forms
First Tender 1971-1972 (12 months)	419.5	63.5	483.0	176	255
Second Tender 1973-1974 (18 months)	745.1	23.8	768.9	222	317
Third Tender 1975-1976 (24 months)	1,219.8	214.6	1,434.4	228	329
Extension of Contracts 1977	—	548.7	548.7	147	—
Fourth Tender 1978-1979 (24 months)	4,322.1	—	4,322.1	181	291
Extension of Contracts 1980 (12 months)	4,363.5	—	4,363.5	51	56

Source: Ministerio de Salud, Oficina Sectorial de Planificacion Evaluacion Socio-Economica.

TABLE 7.2

Sales of Basic Medicines in Peru, 1979–1983
(Millions of 1980 Soles)

Public Sector Institutions	1979		1980		1981		1982		1983		Total	
	Soles	%	Soles	%	Soles	%	Soles	%	Soles	%	Soles	%
Ministry of Health	1,139	32	1,253	39	1,034	45	843	36	279	24	4,548	36
Peruvian Social Security Institute	2,117	60	1,697	53	1,084	47	1,314	57	779	67	6,991	56
Armed Forces and Police	159	5	151	5	101	4	76	3	53	5	540	4
Other Institutions (a)	123	3	117	3	93	4	97	4	44	4	474	4
Total	3,538	100	3,218	100	2,312	100	2,330	100	1,155	100	12,553	100

Note: (a) Cooperatives, clinics, private voluntary organizations, mining companies, municipalities, etc.

Source: Ministerio de Salud, Direccion General de Farmacia, Unidad de Presupuesto y Contabilidad.

TABLE 7.3

Pharmaceutical Suppliers and Their Participation in the Basic Medicines Program in Peru: The 1978-1979 Public Tender (Millions of Current Soles)

	Amount	%
Foreign Pharmaceutical Suppliers		
1. Ifarpe	704.2	
2. Farnac	608.4	
3. Prosalud	259.2	
4. Larpe	216.5	
5. Indufarma	145.5	
6. Eli Lilly Interamericana, Inc.	46.7	
7. Bayer Quimicas Unidas	43.1	
8. Schering Alemana	32.2	
9. Hoechst Peruana	13.2	
10. Cyanamid Peruana	13.0	
11. Upjohn	8.2	
12. Maquifasa	2.3	
Total:	2,092.5	48.5
Local Pharmaceutical Suppliers		
1. Magma	732.0	
2. Laboratorios Unidos	569.6	
3. Efesa	343.9	
4. Farmindustria	212.5	
5. Establecimientos Peruanos Colliere	52.1	
6. Cofana	52.0	
7. Carrion	51.7	
8. Trifarma	26.6	
9. Peikard	23.4	
10. Drogueria Kahan	20.8	
11. Interpharma	18.0	
12. Hersil	12.7	
13. Alfa	5.6	
14. Repasa	3.1	
Total:	2,124.0	49.2
Mixed Pharmaceutical Supplier		
1. Quimica Suiza	98.3	
Total:	98.3	2.3
Grand Total	4,314.8	100.0

Source: Ministerio de Salud, Direccion General de Farmacia.

TABLE 7.4

Quarterly Sales of Essential Medicines in Peru,1984
(Millions of 1980 Soles)

Public Sector Institutions	Quarters, 1984				Total	
	Jan.-Mar.	Apr.-June	July-Sep.	Oct.-Dec.	Soles	Percent
Ministry of Health	103.5	127.9	208.9	197.4	637.7	37
Peruvian Social Security Institute	71.0	127.2	309.0	323.7	830.9	48
Armed Forces and Police	13.6	28.4	86.5	36.1	164.6	9
Other Institutions (a)	7.2	8.7	63.9	26.2	106.0	6
Total	195.3	292.12	668.3	583.4	1,739.2	100

Note: (a) Cooperatives, clinics, private voluntary organizations, mining companies, municipalities, etc.

Source: Ministerio de Salud, Direccion General de Farmacia.

TABLE 7.5

Participation in the National Program of Essential Medicines in Peru, by Type of Firm, 1983
(Millions of 1980 Soles)

	All Participating Firms		Local Firms		Foreign Firms		Mixed Firms	
	Amount	%	Amount	%	Amount	%	Amount	%
Number of firms	25	100	13	52	11	44	1	4
Value of contracts awarded	5,366.9	100	3,635.8	68	1,593.3	30	137.8	2

Source: Ministerio de Salud, Direccion General de Farmacia.

TABLE 7.6

The Pharmaceutical Industry in Latin America, 1980

Country	Pharmaceutical Sales (Millions of US$)	Pharmaceutical Firms (No.)	Market Share of 20 Largest Firms (%)	Market Share of Loc. Owned Firms (%)	Ranking of 4 Largest Locally Owned Firms	Private Sector Sales (% of Total)	Public Sector Sales (% of Total)	Employees (No.)
Argentina	1,920	225	52	47	1,3,10,16	92	8	37,000
Bolivia	32	12	—	NA	NA	50	50	NA
Brazil	1,554	489. (a)	46	22	7,24,30,54	80	20	62,000
Chile	198	41	74	42	1,2,5,14	80	20	5,970
Colombia	560	325	53	12	NA	70	30	15,000
Costa Rica	28	13	82. (c)	18	NA	70	30	NA
Ecuador	96	75	62	11. (b)	1,19,34,49	NA	NA	6,000
Mexico	1,100	315	45	28	31,36,48,51	77	23	43,000
Paraguay	40	24	—	NA	NA	90	10	NA
Peru	200	80	61. (d)	26	4,10,19,27	75	25	17,000
Uruguay	94	69	71	39	10,12,15,18	80	20	2,860
Venezuela	270	75	48	22	2,5,17,23	74	26	7,600

Notes: (a) 1978; (b) 1979; (c) In 1977 just three laboratories accounted for 82% of total production.
(d) The 25 largest pharmaceutical firms.
NA = Not available.

Source: Asociacion Latinoamericana de Industrias Farmaceuticas, "La industria farmaceutica en America Latina: aspectos economicos" (mimeo), October 1981, pp. 12 and 15.

TABLE 7.7

The Peruvian Pharmaceutical Market (Pharmacy Sales):
General Summary, 1977-1984 *

	1977	1978	1979	1980	1981	1982	1983	1984
Total Market								
Units Sold (in thousands)	134,282	119,498	129,742	168,260	140,204	126,787	117,552	105,344
U.S. Dollars (in thousands)	126,129	109,933	124,289	175,779	174,080	159,501	146,369	144,368
Current Soles (in millions)	10,397	15,600	27,203	47,407	71,391	107,297	222,641	483,562
1980 Soles (in millions)	NA	43,212	41,893	47,407	43,549	39,700	37,849	38,685
Ethical Pharmaceuticals								
Units Sold (in thousands)	114,059	101,133	108,703	138,899	120,665	109,940	101,770	92,006
U.S. Dollars (in thousands)	118,129	102,[illegible]4	116,097	164,441	160,518	148,345	136,877	135,228
Current Soles (in millions)	9,740	14,602	25,409	44,353	65,865	99,849	208,216	453,034
1980 Soles (in millions)	NA	40,448	39,130	44,353	40,178	36,944	35,397	36,243
Over-the-Counter Products								
Units Sold (in thousands)	20,223	18,365	21,039	29,361	19,539	16,847	15,782	13,338
U.S. Dollars (in thousands)	8,000	7,029	8,192	11,338	13,562	11,156	9,492	9,140
Current Soles (in millions)	657	998	1,794	3,054	5,526	7,448	14,425	30,528
1980 Soles (in millions)	NA	2,764	2,763	3,054	3,371	2,765	2,452	2,442

* Pharmacy sales account for about 72% of total pharmaceutical sales in Peru.

Source: IMS 1977-84.

TABLE 7.8

Growth Indices for Various Segments of the Peruvian Pharmaceutical Market, 1977-1984
(Pharmacy sales only)

	1977	1978	1979	1980	1981	1982	1983	1984
Total Market								
U.S. Dollars	72	63	71	100	99	91	83	82
Units Sold	80	71	77	100	83	75	70	63
Ethical Pharmaceuticals								
U.S. Dollars	72	63	71	100	98	90	83	82
Units Sold	82	73	78	100	87	79	73	66
Over-the-Counter Products								
U.S. Dollars	71	62	72	100	120	98	84	81
Units Sold	69	63	72	100	67	57	54	45

Source: Derived from Table 7.7.

TABLE 7.9

Unit Price and Per Capita Consumption of Pharmaceuticals in Peru, 1977-1984

	1977	1978	1979	1980	1981	1982	1983	1984
Total Pharmacy Sales *								
U.S. Dollars (thousands)	126,130	109,930	124,290	175,780	174,080	159,500	146,370	144,370
Units (in thousands)	134,280	119,500	129,740	168,260	140,200	126,790	117,550	105,340
Population (in thousands)	15,990	16,414	16,849	17,295	17,755	18,226	18,707	19,198
Average Unit Price (US$)	0.94	0.92	0.96	1.04	1.24	1.26	1.25	1.37
Annual Per Capita Consumption								
U.S. Dollars	7.89	6.70	7.38	10.16	9.80	8.75	7.82	7.52
Units	8.40	7.28	7.70	9.73	7.90	6.96	6.28	5.49

* Pharmacy sales accounted for 71.8% of total pharmaceutical sales in Peru in 1984. Thus the annual per capita consumption figures understate actual consumption by about 30 percent.

Source: International Marketing Service (pharmacy sales) and Instituto Nacional de Estadistica, Lima, Peru (population figures).

TABLE 7.10

Pharmaceutical Prices, Inflation, and Devaluation in Peru, 1976-1983

	Pharmaceutical Prices (a)		Cost-of-living index (b)		Exchange Rate		
Year	Index	Annual Increase	Index (Yearly Average)	Annual Increase	Soles per US$ (Yearly Average)	Annual Index	Increase
1976	100	—	100	—	58	100	—
1977	128	28%	138	38%	87	151	51%
1978	216	69%	218	58%	159	276	83%
1979	315	46%	366	68%	227	395	43%
1980	422	34%	582	59%	293	510	29%
1981	633	50%	1,019	75%	430	750	47%
1982	950	50%	1,671	64%	718	1,253	67%
1983	2,206	132%	3,526	111%	1,639	2,857	128%

Notes: (a) These refer to the average sales prices during each year for 24 pharmaceutical companies included in Price Waterhouse's sample. These companies accounted for around 55 percent of total sales in the Peruvian pharmaceutical industry in 1983.
(b) This index is calculated by the National Institute ofStatistics in Peru.

Source: Price Waterhouse 1984, Tables 13.1 to 13.3.

TABLE 7.11

Nationality and Operating Status of the Principal Pharmaceutical Companies in Peru, 1985

Company	Country of Origin	Has Own Manufacturing Plant	Name of Manufacturer (Own Plant or Contract Manufacturer)
Roche	Switzerland	Yes	Productos Roche Quimica Farmaceutica S.A.
Roussel (a)	West Germany/France	Yes	Laboratorios Larpe S.A.
Farmindustria	National	Yes	Laboratorios Farmindustria S.A.
Schering Corporation	USA	No	Laboratorios Efesa S.A.
Merck Sharp & Dohme	USA	No (e)	Laboratorios Efesa S.A.
Abeefe	National	Yes	Abeefe Laboratorios S.A.
Upjohn	USA	No	Farmitalia Carlo Erba S.A.
Boehringer Ingelheim	West Germany	No	Laboratorios Alfa S.A.
Schering Peruana	West Germany	Yes	Schering Farmaceutica Peruana S.A.
Parke Davis	USA	Yes	Laboratorios Indufarma S.A.
Sandoz	Switzerland	Yes	Sandoz Peru S.A.
Abbott	USA	Yes	Abbott Laboratories S.A.
Squibb	USA	Yes	Manufactureros Quimicos Farmaceuticos S.A. (Maquifasa-Squibb)
Medifarma	National	Yes	Laboratorios Efesa S.A.
Merck S.A.	West Germany	Yes (f)	Laboratorios Cipa S.A.

Grunenthal	West Germany	No	Hoechst Peruana S.A.
Pfizer	USA	Yes	Corporacion Farmaceutica S.A.
Bayer	West Germany	Yes	Bayer Quimicas Unidas S.A.
Merrell	USA	No	Laboratorios Larpe S.A.
Hoechst	West Germany	Yes	Hoechst Peruana S.A
Wyeth	USA	Yes	Laboratorios Wyeth S.A.
Ciba (b)	Switzerland	Yes	Laboratorios Farnac S.A.
Lusa (c)	National	Yes	Laboratorios Unidos S.A.
Winthrop	USA	Yes	Farmaceutica del Pacifico S.A. (Farpasa)
Hersil	National	Yes	Hersil S.A.
Geigy (b)	Switzerland	Yes	Laboratorios Farnac S.A.
Bristol	USA	Yes	Farquimica Andina S.A. (Farquisa)
Carlo Erba	Italy	Yes	Farmitalia Carlo Erba S.A.
Rhone Poulenc	France	No	Laboratorios Alfa S.A.
Lilly	USA	No	Laboratorios Efesa S.A.
Sanitas (d)	National	Yes	Instituto Sanitas S.P. S.A.
Vick	USA	No	Laboratorios Berco S.A.
Cipa	West Germany/Peru	Yes (f)	Laboratorios Cipa S.A.
Pharvet	National	Yes	Laboratorios Pavil S.A.
Atral	Portugal/Peru	Yes	Laboratorios Atral del Peru S.A.

(Continued)

TABLE 7.11 (Cont.)

Company	Country of Origin	Has Own Manufacturing Plant	Name of Manufacturer (Own Plant or Contract Manufacturer)
Magma (d)	National	Yes	Laboratorios Magma S.A.
Trifarma	National	Yes	Laboratorios Trifarma S.A.
Cofana	National	Yes	Consorcio Farmaceutico Nacional
Alfa	National	Yes	Laboratorios Alfa S.A.

Notes: (a) Hoechst (West Germany) acquired a majority interest in Roussel Uclaf (France) in 1976.
(b) A single Swiss firm, Ciba-Geigy, is the parent company of both Ciba and Geigy in Peru.
(c) Lusa is one of two government owned pharmaceutical companies in Peru. The other is Indumil (Industrias Militares).
(d) Sanitas and Magma are both owned by Juan Garrido Pinzon, the son of a former Peruvian senator, Marco Antonio Garrido Malo, whose other son, Gerardo Garrido Pinzon, owns Sintesis Quimica, S.A. (Sinquisa).
(e) In 1984, Merck Sharp ¶ Dohme sold its manufacturing plant (Laboratorios Prosalud S.A.) to Medifarma.
(f) Merck S.A. purchased the majority of the stock in Cipa (Centro de Investigacion Peruano-Argentino) several years ago.

Source: Interviews with company representatives.

8

The Ministry of Health: Financing and Coverage

Dieter K. Zschock

The Peruvian Ministry of Health (MOH) is responsible for providing modern health care for about 11 million medically indigent Peruvians—close to 60 percent of the country's total population. But the current level of MOH funding—equivalent to 27 percent of total health sector expenditures (see Table 1.1)—and the current allocation of these funds provide coverage for only five million inhabitants (see Table 1.3 and Annex B). Moreover, while the MOH has promoted the expansion of primary health care (PHC) as a national policy priority since at least 1980 (Bazan 1985), most of its resources are currently allocated not to this task but to the delivery of hospital care. This long-standing disparity between policy and performance has been exacerbated during Peru's recent severe economic recession.

Between 1980 and 1984, the MOH suffered a 16 percent reduction in expenditures, roughly equivalent to the decline in GDP *per capita* over this period. The Ministry's share of central government expenditures (CGE), however, remained relatively stable at between 4.0 and 4.5 percent between 1980 and 1984, which suggests that the priority assigned to public health did not change significantly. Yet in view of the Peruvian population's increasing impoverishment during the recession, it could be argued that the government should have allocated more resources to public health.

The Ministry's share of total Peruvian health sector expenditures declined only slightly over the period 1980-84 (see Table 1.1). In absolute terms, however, the MOH had only about US $200 million to spend in 1984 compared with some US $235 million annually in 1980 and 1981. Moreover, while the Ministry's financial resources shrank by about 16 percent, Peru's population increased by almost the same percentage. Average *per capita* expenditures for the Ministry's target population of 11 million thus dropped from about US $24 in 1980 to US $20 in 1984. But MOH services are accessible to fewer than half this total. *Per capita* expenditures for the estimated five million people the Ministry does reach are thus twice this average, or about US $40.

This average, however, hides a fundamental misallocation of resources, considering the Ministry's primary health care policy objectives. With over two-thirds of all MOH hospital beds and about the same proportion of medical doctors employed by the MOH located in Peru's major urban areas, home to one-third of the country's population (see Chapters 5 and 6), the Ministry's financial expenditures are also concentrated in the cities. MOH services are within reach of about two million urban and three million rural poor, leaving one million urban and five million rural poor, also dependent on public health care, without access to MOH services.

Primary health care, a Peruvian policy priority since 1980, has presented a particular problem. Because of the urban concentration of MOH hospital facilities and medical personnel, and because of the heavy financial burden that hospital services place on the Ministry, only about one-fourth of total MOH expenditures are used to provide primary health care. This means that the MOH actually spends only about US $10 *per capita*—not US $40—to provide primary health care for the estimated five million urban and rural poor to whom its services are accessible. Since available data on health services utilization do not permit any assessment of the quantitative, and much less the qualitative, adequacy of primary health services, one cannot conclude whether $10 *per capita* is enough, too much, or too little to spend on primary health care, but what circumstantial evidence there is suggests that many MOH health centers and posts are poorly maintained and have insufficient inventories of essential medicines and other supplies (see Chapter 5).

Ministry of Health Expenditures

Revenues vs. Expenditures

Standard budget data obtained from the MOH for the 1980-1984 period allow one to discern some important aspects of its revenues and expenditures, even if they do not permit detailed calculations of expenditures by level of care, types of services, or unit costs of services. For the period 1982-84, Central Government tax revenues declined from 88.5 to 86.7 percent of total MOH income (Table 8.1). User fees also declined, from 8.2 to 7.2 percent. Bearing in mind that financial resources declined in absolute terms, the increase—both proportional and absolute—of borrowing takes on particular significance. Most of this borrowing was foreign aid, although some of the Ministry's deficit was also financed from domestic sources of credit (largely for construction of facilities). All in all, borrowed funds increased from 1.5 to 4.6 percent of total MOH revenues between 1982 and 1984. The source of revenue labeled "transfers" (Table 8.1) includes counterpart funding for foreign aid loans as well as grant aid—if it was received in monetary form; in-kind contributions are not accounted for in MOH budgetary records.

More revealing is the information in Table 8.2, showing the relationship between sources of revenue and expenditures by program category. The MOH budget has identified program areas separately only since 1982; prior to this, all centrally-funded programs were lumped into one category. In addition to "Central Administration" in Table 8.2, the MOH now includes seven central program categories. All health services except for those delivered under these seven centrally-funded and administered programs were financed and administered through the Ministry's 16 health regions as they existed in 1984.

Centrally-funded activities include virtually all facilities construction and the purchase of most equipment ("Physical Facilities"); the construction of rural water and sanitation facilities and the provision of goods and some related services through these facilities ("Environmental Programs"); in-service training of MOH employees ("Training"); the maintenance of a national institute that conducts bio-medical research and tests drugs for consumption in Peru ("National Institute of Health"); and the administration of programs to provide nutritional supplements through health facilities ("Nutrition"). To these five program areas, separately identified as of 1982, two more were added in 1983 and 1984: "Communicable Diseases" and "Primary Health Care."

"Central Administration," which represents close to nine percent of total MOH expenditures, is financed almost entirely by tax revenues. "Physical Facilities" is the next largest expenditure category, representing about seven percent of the total MOH budget; about 40 percent of those expenditures are financed with borrowed funds, with the rest paid for out of tax revenues. The "Nutrition" and "Primary Health Care" programs together account for about six percent of total MOH expenditures; nutrition is largely financed from tax revenues and some user fees, while the primary health care category represents mostly foreign aid and counterpart funding. Normal operating expenditures, including the salaries of primary health care staff, are not included here, but appear in the Ministry's regional line item budget (see below).

All told, central level activities accounted for about 28 percent of total MOH expenditures in 1984—a proportion that had increased substantially from the 1982 level of 23 percent when the effort to regionalize health services administration was initiated. Tax revenues allocated to the MOH during this period declined from 54 billion to 50 billion *soles*, but borrowing tripled, which largely offset the declines in income from general tax revenues and user fees (see Tables 8.1 and 8.2). It is the increase in borrowing (*i.e.*, foreign aid), as well as the increase in the number of centrally-funded and administered programs, that explains the relative increase in central MOH expenditures and the corresponding proportional reductions in regional expenditures.

Despite these reductions, the MOH pursued its policy of regionalizing the administration of health services throughout the 1982-84 period. This policy engendered a major reorganization within the Ministry in 1983, since the administration of health services, which had been carried out at the department level until 1982, now began to be conducted at the level of health regions that no longer coincided with state boundaries. Initially, in 1982, five such regions had been created, but by 1984 this number had been increased to 16, and by 1985 there were 18 separate health regions. All of these have now been eliminated in favor of a much larger number of so-called "local health systems," created under the new government as part of its effort to foster community participation (see Chapter 3).

As the 1982-83 economic recession hit Peru, the MOH tried to soften its impact on recurrent expenditures by sharply curtailing capital spending (Table 8.3) as well as by increasing funding through centrally-funded programs (Table 8.2). The increase was especially notable in the case of the nutrition program, which reached a funding peak in 1983—the year national disasters struck Peru and the recession reached its depth. Overall, recurrent expenditures increased proportionately from 90 percent in 1981 to 94 percent in 1983, and then declined to 90 percent in 1984; they were curtailed more sharply at the central level than the regional, in order to protect regional-level recurrent obligations. Capital spending decreased by half between 1981 and 1983, but recovered in 1984 as foreign aid expenditures increased and economic conditions improved. Increases in capital expenditures administered at the regional level in 1982-83, however, were not sustained in 1984.

Expenditures by Budget Line Items

MOH central expenditures are shown by program in Table 8.4, which provides figures for recurrent and capital spending by line item for each program. It is noteworthy in this table that the central administration budget is heavily burdened by pension payment obligations; that almost two-thirds of the nutrition program consists of expenditures for goods and services, with the balance going for wages; that over three-fourths of environmental program expenditures are for the construction of water ducts and sanitation facilities; and that the PHC program at the central level consists largely of health center and health post construction and the provision of equipment for these facilities, which are financed mostly with foreign aid and required domestic counterpart funds. Wages for MOH central administration represented only six percent of total central MOH expenditures and less than two percent of the total MOH budget that year. It cannot be said, therefore, that the MOH is top-heavy with administrative costs. Instead, the MOH exerts its still very much centralized power through its control of expenditures for goods and services and for the financing of construction and equipment purchases. The "Pensions" category provides further evidence of the Ministry's administrative centralization.

Table 8.5, in which the evolution of MOH total recurrent expenditures over the five-year period from 1980-84 is shown, illustrates the recent growth in the proportion of wages and benefits as well as pension payments. Even as the Ministry's total resources were shrinking by 16 percent, its expenditures for wages and benefits were increasing, in real terms, by nine percent—from 33 million *soles* in 1980 to 36 million in 1984. Wages actually topped 38 billion *soles* in 1983, the year of economic and natural catastrophes. Pension payments also doubled, in both relative and absolute terms, and now account for nine percent of total MOH recurrent expenditures annually. This expansion in personnel expenditures was clearly irresponsible, particularly in light of the sharp reduction in expenditures for goods and services, the two line items that include essential medicines and other supplies as well as maintenance. Purchases of goods declined from 15.3 billion *soles* in 1981 to 8.7 billion in 1984—*i.e.*, from 24 to 17 percent of total recurrent expenditures.

Transfer payments also fell victim to the Ministry's protection of its wage and pension budgets. The reduction of transfers from 11 to just over one percent of total recurrent expenditures is particularly significant, since the Ministry formerly supported health services provided by private voluntary organizations (PVOs) under this budget item. MOH protection of its recurrent cost obligations, especially at the regional level where most of its wage expenditures are concentrated, has coincided with the virtual elimination of support for PVOs (which mostly provide much-needed primary health care) and a sharp reduction in the goods and services that are essential to the provision of primary health care in the public sector. The only increases in spending have been for PHC facilities and for the wages of medical personnel to staff them.

Buildings and staff, however, do not add up to effective primary health care delivery in the absence of maintenance and medicines. Table 8.6, outlining MOH capital expenditures, shows that these declined, in absolute terms, by over 50 percent—from 9.4 billion *soles* in 1980 to 6.0 billion in 1984. The major reduction in capital spending was in construction; purchases of equipment (most of it provided through foreign aid) actually increased. While the increase in equipment purchases was undoubtedly necessary, the reduction in construction has had mixed effects. New hospital construction has been slowed significantly—a positive development, since the MOH is excessively burdened by hospital costs and oversupplied with beds (see Chapter 5). Renovation of existing health centers and posts and of regional hospitals, however, came to a virtual standstill. This, together with an almost total lack of expenditures for maintenance, has led to a serious decline in the serviceability of many of the Ministry's ambulatory and inpatient facilities, particularly outside the Lima/Callao metropolitan area.

Expenditures at the Regional Level

A comparison of MOH central and regional level expenditures shows that goods, services, and pensions dominate the composition of the recurrent budget at the central level, while wages and benefits account for most of the recurrent expenditures at the regional level (Tables 8.7 to 8.10). Moreover, almost all capital expenditures are made at the central level. These observations suggest that the Ministry's much-touted regionalization of health services administration has not actually resulted in reductions of control over the most important and most volatile variable expenditures: the purchase of goods, services, and equipment and the construction and renovation of facilities. The Ministry remained a highly centralized organization, despite the fact that 73 percent of its budget in 1984 was administered by the health regions (Table 8.3).

The absolute growth in wage and benefit expenditures at the regional level, particularly since this occurred during a period of severe economic recession, appears to be related to the regionalization of health services administration. However, it has not been possible to determine to what extent this growth was due, respectively, to wage increases and employment expansion.

One of the objectives of the regionalization of health services administration has been to redress the considerable imbalance in the allocation of MOH resources. But in the three years from 1982 to 1984, during which regionalization was implemented, the shares of financing for which the 16 health regions accounted did not change significantly (Table 8.11). Lima/Callao's share declined from 48.9 to 47.9 percent, and the five southern Andean regions—Puno, Cusco, Ayacucho, Huancayo, and Huanuco—increased their combined share from 17.7 to 18.4 percent. These five regions have been singled out for support under the government's PHC policy. The country's poorest regions in the north—Piura, Chiclayo, and Cajamarca—suffered a decline in their combined share of MOH financing from 8.8 to 8.5 percent. The fact that these were the regions hardest hit by natural disasters in 1983 may have lessened their absorptive capacity for expenditures by the Ministry, even if they needed more rather than less support.

The wages and benefits share of regional expenditures, which averaged 79 percent in 1984, varied considerably among regions (Table 8.12). It was almost identical to the national average in the three most urbanized regions (Lima/Callao, Ica, and Arequipa), highest in the poorest regions (such as

Cajamarca and Puno), and slightly below the national average in most of the other regions. The larger a region's share of wages and benefits, of course, the lower its share of essential medicines and other supplies, and also of services such as maintenance.

The category "Other" in Table 8.12 is broken down into some of its major components in Table 8.13. Here the all-too-small proportions of regional-level health care expenditures allocated to medicines and maintenance are evident. In a reasonably well-supplied health service, medicines would account for approximately 15 percent of total expenditures, but the average for all Peruvian health regions is only 5.2 percent. Only two regions—Ayacucho and Huancayo—significantly exceeded the national average for expenditures for both medicines and maintenance; the majority of the regions had even less to spend on medicines and maintenance than the national average. Not even the three urban regions were substantially better supplied with these essential goods and services.

The extent of the inequality in the distribution of MOH resources among the 16 health regions is evident in Table 8.14, which compares their population shares with their shares of total regional expenditures, hospital beds, and health centers and posts. These data allow one to determine to what extent the distribution of financial resources is a function of population distribution (as it probably should be), the distribution of secondary and tertiary care (hospital beds), or the distribution of primary care facilities (health centers and posts).

It is obvious that the distribution of both expenditures and hospital beds strongly favors the Lima/Callao health region, whose 28 percent of the country's population benefits from almost half of these resources. The imbalance between primary and secondary/tertiary levels of care in this metropolitan area is also apparent. With approximately 20 percent of the country's medically indigent population, Lima/Callao has only 13 percent of all primary care facilities, which helps to explain why hospital-based ambulatory services are so heavily utilized for primary care in the capital (HSA-Peru 1986c). In the rest of the country, health centers and posts are more evenly distributed in relation to population. However, econometric analysis of the data in Table 8.14 suggests that regional financial shares are more likely a function of the regions' hospital bedshares than of their primary care facility shares (1).

There are probably many other variables that influence the distribution of health care expenditures. The fact that the distribution of primary health care facilities does not significantly affect the allocation of financial resources by region (and may even be negatively related to expenditures) suggests that the Ministry's PHC policy priority has had no bearing on how it has actually distributed its financial resources. This finding is also supported by evidence that over half of all health centers and posts outside the major urban areas may be inoperative due to poor maintenance (see Chapter 5). While primary health care facilities appear to have been built in some relationship to population distribution, econometric analysis does not support this as a statistically significant relationship (2).

In other words, neither population nor the distribution of primary health care facilities has had any apparent impact on how the MOH has distributed its financial resources among health regions. The quantitative analysis suggests that other variables are more important in the distribution of primary health care facilities than these seemingly most obvious ones, but it is not apparent what those other variables might be.

The conclusion that MOH regionalization of health services has not improved the efficiency of PHC delivery is supported by analyses of financial and services administration carried out by a Peruvian group under contract to the country's Central Bank and the World Bank (de Arregui *et al.* 1985), and by a US Agency for International Health contract firm (Westinghouse 1985). These analyses show that decision-making about resources allocation has remained concentrated at the central MOH level, that there has been little improvement in administrative capabilities at the regional level, and that PHC facilities have remained seriously understaffed, poorly maintained, and insufficiently supplied with medicines and other supplies.

Foreign technical assistance for MOH management improvement (see below) was largely frustrated by the instability of leadership at the regional level between 1983 and 1985. It is not surprising then that—given the reductions in MOH financial resources and regional leadership instability—concern over wages and benefits among MOH administrators and health service staff took precedence over the need to increase the availability of medicines and other essential goods and services to primary health care facilities.

Foreign Aid Contributions

Over the period 1980-84, the MOH spent approximately US $1.1 billion, for an average of $220 million annually (see Table 1.1). Five major sources of foreign aid accounted for the equivalent of about four percent of this total. The Pan American Health Organization (PAHO), the World Bank, the Interamerican Development Bank (IDB), and the US (USAID) and West German (GTZ) bilateral foreign aid programs together made available about U.S. $70 million (Table 8.15). Two-thirds of this total represented low-interest loan funds with long repayment periods; the other one-third was in the form of grant funds. However, the largest loan—US $33.5 from the World Bank—has remained largely unused, meaning that only about $40 million in foreign aid was actually expended over the five-year period.

Disbursement of foreign aid—particularly of USAID funds—was slow in the initial years, but was accelerated from 1983 onward. Of the foreign aid actually used by the MOH (that is, excluding the World Bank loan), USAID contributions represented over 70 percent, or a total of $29 million. Two-thirds of the USAID contribution has been in the form of loan funds, which have been used primarily for expenditures on equipment, transportation, supplies, training, and technical assistance at the primary health care level. These funds show up in the MOH budget (see above) as revenue generated through borrowing. The remaining one-third of the USAID contribution, in grant funds, has been used primarily to pay for technical assistance, as well as some supplies and training to complement the MOH loan-funded assistance program. Only those grant funds actually transferred to the MOH appear in its budget, under "transfers."

Both the PAHO and IDB grants represented funds transferred to the MOH. The GTZ grant, like those from USAID, was split between technical assistance and goods and services. Again, only transfers of funds, not contributions in kind, appear in the MOH budget as revenue. While no exact calculations of total financial contributions are possible, one can conclude that in reality these represented, on the average, no more than three percent of MOH revenue over the 1980-84 period. Technical assistance was devoted, to a considerable extent, to helping the MOH make efficient use of the direct contributions of financial and in-kind resources.

To supplement their direct contributions of resources, donor agencies (except PAHO) require the government of Peru to match these resources, at varying ratios, with domestically generated counterpart funds. The intent is to encourage the country to boost its own resources allocated for health care, rather than becoming dependent on foreign aid. To a large extent, however, the government's counterpart funds are generated through another source of foreign aid: revenues from the sale in Peru of US food surpluses. These revenues provide a major source of Peruvian counterpart funding not only for USAID but also for World Bank and IDB contributions.

It is probably impossible to determine whether Peruvian counterpart payments in fact represent a net increase in domestic financing of MOH programs. Likewise, it is difficult to say whether or not foreign aid funds and in-kind transfers represent net additions to domestic financing of health services. To some extent, both counterpart funds and foreign aid contributions probably displace funds from ordinary sources, such as tax revenues and user payments, as well as domestic borrowing for health sector investment expenditures that might otherwise be allocated to the MOH by the Central Government. Considering, in addition, the difficulties imposed on the MOH by foreign aid administrative requirements, one cannot conclude that donors have made a significant financial contribution to the health sector in Peru in recent years.

To discern any positive impact foreign aid may have had on the Peruvian health sector, one must assess how it has encouraged and enabled Peruvian authorities to implement significant changes in the orientation of MOH services. Certainly primary health care is now accorded financing priority, in that a separate budget category, for which close to 10 percent of total MOH expenditures (excluding recurrent labor costs) are earmarked, has been created to channel resources directly for this purpose. However, this category consists largely of investment expenditures (facilities, equipment, training) funded by foreign aid and counterpart monies. Operating expenditures—particularly the wages and benefits of primary health care workers, plus medicine, maintenance, etc.—are still encompassed within the respective budgetary line items of the Ministry.

It is therefore impossible, on the basis of MOH budgetary records, to determine with any accuracy how much the Ministry spends on primary health care. The conclusion that 25 percent of total MOH spending, at best, has been devoted to PHC must remain a "ball park" estimate. This 25 percent figure in turn represents between six and seven percent of total health sector expenditures. Despite being unable to state exactly how much—either in absolute terms or in proportion to total available health sector spending—should be allocated to the 11 million Peruvians who depend heavily on the MOH for health care delivery, it seems clear that 25 percent of the Ministry's budget is not enough.

It is also worth noting that the MOH would have suffered sharper budgetary reductions over the period 1982-84 were it not for a growing influx of foreign aid since 1980. The expenditure data suggest a clear correspondence between the Peruvian government's waning commitment to the MOH between 1980 and 1984 and its acceptance of substantially increased foreign donor support for primary health care.

Conclusions

Total health sector expenditures in Peru are at a level compatible with the country's level of economic development, but a third of the population—predominantly in the rural areas—has no financial and/or geographical access to modern health care. There is an inherent policy conflict, however, between the economically stronger urban areas and the underdeveloped rural areas of Peru. Both need and demand more and better health care, but while health sector leaders have paid lip service to the priority of primary health care during the past five years, they have continued to allocate the large majority of financial, physical, and human resources to secondary and tertiary level care in the large urban centers. Donors of foreign aid have supported the expansion of primary health care, but the Peruvian government has not been able or willing to reorient its own spending priorities to match its policy priorities in the health sector.

In addition to these observations, the following specific conclusions can be drawn from the analysis presented here:

1. The Ministry of Health, which by law is responsible for the health care of all medically indigent Peruvians, provided coverage (in 1984) for about five million people—two million in towns and cities and three million in rural areas. An estimated six million medically indigent Peruvians were left without coverage—one million in urban and five million in rural areas. This disparity between mandated and actual population coverage is a result more of the actual distribution of MOH resources than its overall level of financial support.

2. The percentage of health sector financing the Ministry of Health commands—slightly more than a quarter of total expenditures for the sector—is roughly equal to the share of the population it currently covers and to the percentage of medical doctors it employs. However, its financing percentage is grossly unequal to the percentage of PHC facilities it operates (86 percent of the country's total), the number of hospital beds it administers (nearly 60 percent of the country's total), and the number of pharmacies it operates (only 10 percent of the total). This suggests that the MOH should either receive substantially more financial support or significantly decrease the number of hospitals for which it is financially responsible.

3. Despite its policy commitment to primary health care, secondary and tertiary health services absorb about three-fourths of MOH financing. The Ministry's PHC program accounts for the remaining one-fourth, and is being provided at about US $10 *per capita* of estimated coverage. This is probably insufficient. A large proportion of PHC facilities are poorly maintained and inadequately staffed. Moreover, they lack essential medicines; even medically indigent Peruvians must buy most of their medicines from private pharmacies. Increased financial support, or reduced financial responsibility for hospitals, should allow the MOH to align its actions more closely with its policy intent.

4. Quantitative analysis indicates that MOH financial allocations are largely determined by the distribution of secondary and tertiary facilities, rather than by population distribution or even the location of primary health care facilities. The relatively equitable distribution (but insufficient total number) of health centers and posts, shown in Chapter 5, is undermined by serious shortages of operating support. Thus, before it can hope to expand primary health care coverage, the MOH needs to rectify current deficiencies in financing the operating costs of already-existing PHC facilities.

5. Despite declining financial resources, MOH expenditures for personnel and benefits, including pensions, increased over the 1980-84 period, to the detriment of facilities maintenance and pharmaceuticals, whose shares of total MOH expenditures have shrunk to such low levels that the delivery of services,

particularly at the primary care level, is now seriously deficient even for the currently covered population. The MOH thus needs to accept responsibility for maintaining an appropriate balance in the allocation of its financial resources among wages, facilities maintenance, supplies, and other critical elements of effective PHC services delivery.

6. The attempts of the MOH to regionalize the administration of its services in order to make them more accessible to its target population have not been effective. The regionalization program has undergone repeated changes over the past five years, yet there has been no effective delegation of responsibility and authority, particularly in the area of financial decision-making. Delegation of responsibility from central to regional levels can work effectively only if sufficient resources, together with the authority to use these resources flexibly but within an agreed-upon policy context, are made available.

Footnotes

1. A regression of the three independent variables (the shares of population, hospital beds, and health centers/posts) on the dependent variable (financial share) shows population to have virtually no impact on the distribution of expenditures (see Table 8.14). Hospital beds, on the other hand, strongly influence financial allocations by region. The regression results are:

$$\text{FINSHARE} = \underset{(t=-0.1)}{\text{Constant }(-309.348)} + \underset{(t=1.8)}{\text{POPSHARE }(0.007)}$$

$$+ \underset{(t=12.8)}{\text{BEDSHARE }(27.361)} - \underset{(t=-0.6)}{\text{HCPSHARE }(16.271)}$$

$R^2 = 0.9$

2. The regression results are:

$$\text{HCPSHARE} = \underset{(t=8.0)}{\text{Constant }(85.221)} - \underset{(t=-0.6)}{\text{FINSHARE }(-0.0)}$$

$$+ \underset{(t=1.8)}{\text{POPSHARE }(0.0)}$$

$R^2 = 0.6$

TABLE 8.1

MOH Sources of Revenue, 1980–84 *

(in billions of current soles)

	1980		1981		1982		1983		1984	
	Total	%	Total	%	Total	%	Total	%	Total	%
All Sources	49.0	100.0	83.2	100.0	166.3	100.0	341.5	100.0	725.6	100.0
Tax Revenue	43.6	89.0	75.5	90.7	147.2	88.5	301.0	88.2	628.9	86.7
User Charges	3.3	6.7	5.2	6.3	13.7	8.2	24.2	7.1	52.1	7.2
Borrowing	1.9	3.9	2.3	2.8	2.4	1.5	9.7	2.8	33.4	4.6
Transfers	0.2	0.4	0.2	0.2	3.0	1.8	6.6	1.9	11.2	1.5

(in billions of 1980 soles)

All Sources	49.0	100.0	50.8	100.0	61.5	100.0	58.1	100.0	58.0	100.0
Tax Revenue	43.6	89.0	46.0	90.7	54.4	88.5	51.2	88.2	50.3	86.7
User Charges	3.3	6.7	3.2	6.3	5.1	8.2	4.1	7.1	4.1	7.2
Borrowing	1.9	3.9	1.5	2.8	0.9	1.5	1.7	2.8	2.7	4.6
Transfers	0.2	0.4	0.1	0.2	1.1	1.8	1.1	1.9	0.9	1.5

Data from MOH budget office records.

* Sources of revenues for final expenditures.

Note: Data for 1980 and 1981 do not include revenues expended for health by the ORDES (state-level development agencies), whose sources are not known.

TABLE 8.2

MOH Expenditures by Source and Program, 1980 - 84
(in millions of 1980 soles)

	CENTRAL LEVEL									
	Central Administration		Training		Physical Facilities		Nat'l Inst. of Health		Nutrition	
	Total	%	Total	%	Total	%	Total	%	Total	%
1980, total	9,349	100.0							15,132	
Tax revenue	9,021	96.5								
User charges	10	0.1								
Borrowing	253	2.7								
Transfers	65	0.7								
1981, total	8,161	100.0							13,552	
Tax revenue	7,835	96.0								
User charges	1	0.0								
Borrowing	310	3.8								
Transfers	16	0.2								
1982, total	4,612	100.0	84	100.0	4,093	100.0	729	100.0	3,475	100.0
Tax revenue	4,160	90.2	83	98.2	2,771	67.7	569	78.0	2,886	83.0
User charges	224	4.9	1	1.8	14	0.4	161	22.0	589	17.0
Borrowing	134	2.9	0	0.0	696	17.0	0	0.0	0	0.0
Transfers	94	2.0	0	0.0	611	14.9	0	0.0	0	0.0
1983, total	4,619	100.0	0		2,814	100.0	776	100.0	3,515	100.0
Tax revenue	4,230	91.6	0		1,490	53.0	539	69.4	3,140	89.3
User charges	139	3.0	0		3	0.1	237	30.6	376	10.7
Borrowing	152	3.3	0		980	34.8	0	0.0	0	0.0
Transfers	98	2.1	0		341	12.1	0	0.0	0	0.0
1984, total	5,162	100.0	61	100.0	4,295	100.0	711	100.0	2,176	100.0
Tax revenue	5,002	96.9	57	93.9	2,560	59.6	553	77.8	1,935	88.9
User charges	140	2.7	4	6.1	4	0.1	156	21.9	240	11.1
Borrowing	0	0.0	0	0.0	1,707	39.8	0	0.0	0	0.0
Transfers	11	0.2	0	0.0	23	0.5	2	0.3	0	0.0

Note: Data from MOH budget office records, except that 1980 and 1981 health region expenditures include funds provided through the ORDES which are not included in MOH records. In later years, all regional funds came from MOH directly.

Environmental Programs		Transmissible Diseases		Primary Health Care		SUBTOTAL		HEALTH REGIONS		MOH TOTALS	
Total	%	Total	%	Total	%	Total	%	Total	%	Total	%
						24,481	100.0	42,745	100.0	67,226	100.0
						21,713	100.0	46,972	100.0	68,685	100.0
932	100.0	0		0		13,925	100.0	47,612	100.0	61,537	100.0
599	64.2	0		0		11,067	79.5	43,386	91.1	54,453	88.5
33	3.5	0		0		1,023	7.3	4,050	8.5	5,073	8.2
77	8.3	0		0		907	6.5	0	0.0	907	1.5
224	24.0	0		0		929	6.7	175	0.4	1,104	1.8
1,053	100.0	1,226	100.0	0		14,002	100.0	44,058	100.0	58,060	100.0
439	41.7	808	65.9	0		10,644	76.0	40,533	92.0	51,177	88.2
48	4.6	0	0.0	0		803	5.7	3,307	7.5	4,110	7.1
279	26.5	239	19.5	0		1,649	11.8	0	0.0	1,649	2.8
287	27.2	179	14.6	0		905	6.5	218	0.5	1,124	1.9
1,129	100.0	926	100.0	1,406	100.0	15,865	100.0	42,179	100.0	58,045	100.0
457	40.5	926	100.0	236	16.8	11,727	73.9	38,582	91.5	50,309	86.7
36	3.2	0	0.0	0	0.0	581	3.7	3,590	8.5	4,171	7.2
396	35.1	0	0.0	570	40.6	2,674	16.9	0	0.0	2,674	4.6
240	21.2	0	0.0	600	42.6	876	5.5	7	0.0	883	1.5

TABLE 8.3

MOH Recurrent and Capital Expenditures by Central and Regional Levels, 1980 - 84
(in millions of 1980 soles)

Category	1980		1981		1982		1983		1984	
	Total	%	Total	%	Total	%	Total	%	Total	%
Total	67,266	100.0	68,685	100.0	61,537	100.0	58,059	100.0	58,044	100.0
Central level	24,481	36.4	21,713	31.6	13,926	22.6	14,001	24.1	15,952	27.5
Regional level	42,745	63.5	46,972	68.4	47,611	77.4	44,058	75.9	42,092	72.5
Recurrent	57,823	86.0	61,628	89.7	56,024	91.0	54,638	94.1	52,001	89.6
Central level	15,732	27.2	14,821	24.0	9,287	16.6	10,896	19.9	10,119	19.5
Regional level	42,091	72.8	46,807	76.0	46,737	83.4	43,742	80.1	41,882	80.5
Capital	9,403	14.0	7,057	10.3	5,513	9.0	3,421	5.9	6,043	10.4
Central level	8,749	93.0	6,892	97.7	4,639	84.1	3,105	90.8	5,833	96.5
Regional level	654	7.0	165	2.3	874	15.9	316	9.2	210	3.5

Data from MOH budget office records.
Note: Central and regional level percentages of respective category totals.

TABLE 8.4

Composition of MOH Central Expenditures by Program Category and Line Item, 1984
(vertical percentages)

	CENTRAL MOH PROGRAMS							
Category and Line Item	Central Admin.	Training	Physical Facilities	Nat'l Inst. of Health	Nutrition	Environmental Programs	Transmissible Diseases	Primary Health Care
Recurrent Expenditure:								
Wages & benefits	19.87	76.20	8.26	53.03	36.89	16.86	8.55	4.09
Goods	2.73	4.63	4.79	14.82	52.88	1.57	64.38	3.02
Services	3.21	5.57	4.12	8.05	10.21	2.65	27.07	1.10
Transfers	13.27	11.83	0.00	0.03	0.02	0.00	0.00	0.25
Pensions	59.99	0.00	0.00	17.11	0.00	0.00	0.00	0.00
Capital Expenditure:								
Studies	0.00	0.00	4.19	0.00	0.00	0.00	0.00	1.32
Construction	0.00	0.00	32.50	0.40	0.00	77.33	0.00	74.59
Equipment	0.00	1.77	46.14	6.50	0.00	1.59	0.00	15.63
Other	0.93	0.00	0.00	0.06	0.00	0.00	0.00	0.00
Total	100.00	100.00	100.00	100.00	100.00	100.00	100.00	100.00

Data from MOH budget office records.

TABLE 8.5

MOH Total Recurrent Expenditures by Line Item, 1980 - 84
(in millions of 1980 soles)

	1980		1981		1982		1983		1984	
Line Item	Total	%	Total	%	Total	%	Total	%	Total	%
Total recurrent expenditures	57,823	100.0	61,628	100.0	56,024	100.0	54,638	100.0	52,001	100.0
Wages & benefits	33,258	57.5	36,109	58.6	39,207	70.0	38,546	70.6	36,217	69.7
Goods	13,866	24.0	15,269	24.8	11,874	21.2	9,901	18.1	8,654	16.6
Services	1,878	3.3	2,373	3.9	1,980	3.5	2,622	4.8	1,880	3.6
Transfers	6387	11.0	5576	9.0	918	1.6	674	1.2	727	1.4
Pensions	2,434	4.2	2,301	3.7	2,045	3.7	2,895	5.3	4,523	8.7

Data from MOH budget office records.

TABLE 8.6

MOH Total Capital Expenditures by Line Item, 1980 - 84
(in millions of 1980 soles)

	1980		1981		1982		1983		1984	
Line Item	Total	%	Total	%	Total	%	Total	%	Total	%
Total capital expenditures	9,403	100.0	7,057	100.0	5,513	100.0	3,421	100.0	6,043	100.0
Studies	256	2.7	253	3.6	195	3.5	47	1.4	199	3.3
Construction	7,940	84.4	5,754	81.5	4,549	82.5	2,199	64.3	3,439	56.9
Equipment	808	8.6	864	12.3	769	14.0	1,150	33.6	2,357	39.0
Other	399	4.3	186	2.6	0	0.0	25	0.7	48	0.8

Data from MOH budget office records.

TABLE 8.7

MOH Recurrent Expenditures by Line Item
Central Level, 1980 - 84
(in millions of 1980 soles)

	1980		1981		1982		1983		1984	
Line Item	Total	%	Total	%	Total	%	Total	%	Total	%
Total	15,732	100.0	14,821	100.0	9,287	100.0	10,896	100.0	10,119	100.0
Wages & benefits	3,336	21.2	4,018	27.1	3,757	40.5	3,427	31.4	2,933	29.0
Goods	5,787	36.8	5,385	36.3	2,525	27.2	3,112	28.6	2,349	23.2
Services	847	5.4	840	5.7	534	5.7	1,543	14.2	903	8.9
Transfers	3,978	25.3	2,955	19.9	901	9.7	668	6.1	716	7.1
Pensions	1,784	11.3	1,623	11.0	1,570	16.9	2,146	19.7	3,218	31.8

Data from MOH budget office records.

TABLE 8.8

MOH Capital Expenditures by Line Item
Central Level, 1980 - 84
(in millions of 1980 soles)

	1980		1981		1982		1983		1984	
Line Item	Total	%	Total	%	Total	%	Total	%	Total	%
Total	8,749	100.0	6,892	100.0	4,639	100.0	3,105	100.0	5,833	100.0
Studies	256	2.9	253	3.7	195	4.2	47	1.5	199	3.4
Construction	7,657	87.5	5,638	81.8	4,232	91.2	2,102	67.7	3,439	59.0
Equipment	437	5.0	815	11.8	212	4.6	931	30.0	2,147	36.8
Other	399	4.6	186	2.7	0	0.0	25	0.8	48	0.8

Data from MOH budget office records.

TABLE 8.9

MOH Recurrent Expenditures by Line Item, Regional Level, 1980 - 84
(in millions of 1980 soles)

	1980		1981		1982		1983		1984	
Line Item	Total	%	Total	%	Total	%	Total	%	Total	%
Total	42,091	100.0	46,807	100.0	46,737	100.0	43,742	100.0	41,882	100.0
Wages & benefits	29,922	71.1	32,091	68.6	35,450	75.9	35,119	80.3	33,284	79.5
Goods	8,079	19.2	9,884	21.1	9,349	20.0	6,789	15.5	6,305	15.1
Services	1,031	2.5	1,533	3.3	1,446	3.1	1,079	2.5	977	2.3
Transfers	2,409	5.7	2,621	5.6	17	0.0	6	0.0	11	0.0
Pensions	650	1.5	678	1.4	475	1.0	749	1.7	1,305	3.1

Data from MOH budget office records

TABLE 8.10

MOH Capital Expenditures by Line Item,
Regional Level, 1980 - 84
(in millions of 1980 soles)

	1980		1981		1982		1983		1984	
Line Item	Total	%	Total	%	Total	%	Total	%	Total	%
Total	654	100.0	165	100.0	874	100.0	316	100.0	210	100.0
Studies	0	0.0	0	0.0	0	0.0	0	0.0	0	0.0
Construction	283	43.3	116	70.3	317	36.3	97	30.7	0	0.0
Equipment	371	56.7	49	29.7	557	63.7	219	69.3	210	100.0
Other	0	0.0	0	0.0	0	0.0	0	0.0	0	0.0

Data from MOH budget office records

TABLE 8.11

Distribution of Total MOH Regional Expenditures, 1982 - 84
(in millions of 1980 soles)

	1982		1983		1984	
Region	Total	%	Total	%	Total	%
Piura	1,913	4.0	1,655	3.8	1,583	3.8
Chiclayo	1,559	3.3	1,371	3.1	1,338	3.2
Cajamarca	716	1.5	629	1.4	638	1.5
Trujillo	2,301	4.8	2,175	4.9	2,115	5.0
Huaraz	1,621	3.4	1,787	4.1	1,563	3.7
Lima/Callao	23,259	48.9	21,762	49.4	20,207	47.9
Ica	2,004	4.2	1,812	4.1	1,665	3.9
Arequipa	2,498	5.2	2,524	5.7	2,305	5.5
Tacna	1,186	2.5	1,062	2.4	1,058	2.5
Puno	1,215	2.6	1,178	2.7	1,315	3.1
Cusco	2,334	4.9	1,963	4.5	2,001	4.7
Ayacucho	734	1.5	591	1.3	611	1.4
Huancayo	2,618	5.5	2,403	5.5	2,573	6.1
Huanuco	1,507	3.2	1,257	2.9	1,320	3.1
Moyobamba	1,092	2.3	967	2.2	1,008	2.4
Iquitos	1,054	2.2	922	2.1	879	2.1
Total	47,611	100.0	44,058	100.0	42,179	100.0

Data from MOH budget office records.

Note: Chiclayo is Lambayeque-Amazonas region.

TABLE 8.12

Share of Wage Expenditures in MOH Total Regional Expenditures, 1982 - 84

(in millions of 1980 soles and horizontal distribution in percentages)

	1982					
Region	Wages	%	Other	%	Total	%
Piura	1,557	81.4	356	18.6	1,913	100.0
Chiclayo	1,325	85.0	234	15.0	1,559	100.0
Cajamarca	538	75.1	178	24.9	716	100.0
Trujillo	1,952	84.8	349	15.2	2,301	100.0
Huaraz	1,298	80.1	323	19.9	1,621	100.0
Lima/Callao	16,555	71.2	6,704	28.8	23,259	100.0
Ica	1,624	81.0	380	19.0	2,004	100.0
Arequipa	2,031	81.3	467	18.7	2,498	100.0
Tacna	883	74.5	303	25.5	1,186	100.0
Puno	972	80.0	243	20.0	1,215	100.0
Cusco	1,782	76.3	552	23.7	2,334	100.0
Ayacucho	518	70.6	216	29.4	734	100.0
Huancayo	1,812	69.2	806	30.8	2,618	100.0
Huanuco	1,016	67.4	491	32.6	1,507	100.0
Moyobamba	744	68.1	348	31.9	1,092	100.0
Iquitos	843	80.0	211	20.0	1,054	100.0
Total	35,450	74.5	12,161	25.5	47,611	100.0

(Continued)

TABLE 8.12 (Cont.)

	1983					
Region	Wages	%	Other	%	Total	%
Piura	1,364	82.4	291	17.6	1,655	100.0
Chiclayo	1,221	89.1	150	10.9	1,371	100.0
Cajamarca	486	77.3	143	22.7	629	100.0
Trujillo	1,847	84.9	328	15.1	2,175	100.0
Huaraz	1,330	74.4	457	25.6	1,787	100.0
Lima/Callao	17,094	78.5	4,668	21.5	21,762	100.0
Ica	1,540	85.0	272	15.0	1,812	100.0
Arequipa	2,087	82.7	437	17.3	2,524	100.0
Tacna	815	76.7	247	23.3	1,062	100.0
Puno	1,010	85.7	168	14.3	1,178	100.0
Cusco	1,536	78.2	427	21.8	1,963	100.0
Ayacucho	437	73.9	154	26.1	591	100.0
Huancayo	1,819	75.7	584	24.3	2,403	100.0
Huanuco	932	74.1	325	25.9	1,257	100.0
Moyobamba	691	71.5	276	28.5	967	100.0
Iquitos	728	79.0	194	21.0	922	100.0
Total	34,937	79.3	9,121	20.7	44,058	100.0

TABLE 8.12 (Cont.)

	1984					
Region	Wages	%	Other	%	Total	%
Piura	1,265	79.9	318	20.1	1,583	100.0
Chiclayo	1,152	86.1	186	13.9	1,338	100.0
Cajamarca	509	79.8	129	20.2	638	100.0
Trujillo	1,689	79.9	426	20.1	2,115	100.0
Huaraz	1,293	82.7	270	17.3	1,563	100.0
Lima/Callao	16,069	79.5	4,138	20.5	20,207	100.0
Ica	1,350	81.1	315	18.9	1,665	100.0
Arequipa	1,824	79.1	481	20.9	2,305	100.0
Tacna	785	74.2	273	25.8	1,058	100.0
Pun	1,139	86.6	176	13.4	1,315	100.0
Cusco	1,561	78.0	440	22.0	2,001	100.0
Ayacucho	451	73.8	160	26.2	611	100.0
Huancayo	1,809	70.3	764	29.7	2,573	100.0
Huanuco	966	73.2	354	26.8	1,320	100.0
Moyobamba	748	74.2	260	25.8	1,008	100.0
Iquitos	674	76.7	205	23.3	879	100.0
Total	33,284	78.9	8,895	21.1	42,179	100.0

Data from MOH budget office records.

Note: Chiclayo is Lambayeque-Amazonas region.

TABLE 8.13

Comparison of MOH Total Regional Expenditures Between Wages and Selected Goods and Services, 1984

(in millions of 1980 soles and horizontal distribution in percentages)

	Wages		Medicines		Lab. Supplies	
Region	Total	%	Total	%	Total	%
Piura	1,265	79.9	51	3.2	5	0.3
Chiclayo	1,152	86.1	21	1.6	2	0.1
Cajamarca	509	79.8	36	5.6	1	0.2
Trujillo	1,689	79.9	69	3.3	11	0.5
Huaraz	1,293	82.7	58	3.7	4	0.3
Lima/Callao	16,069	79.5	1,137	5.6	145	0.7
Ica	1,350	81.1	50	3.0	5	0.3
Arequipa	1,824	79.1	46	2.0	4	0.2
Tacna	785	74.2	61	5.8	2	0.2
Puno	1,139	86.6	46	3.5	3	0.2
Cusco	1,561	78.0	90	4.5	6	0.3
Ayacucho	451	73.8	70	11.5	6	1.0
Huancayo	1,809	70.3	263	10.2	16	0.6
Huanuco	966	73.2	109	8.3	6	0.5
Moyobamba	748	74.2	85	8.4	4	0.4
Iquitos	674	76.7	11	1.3	1	0.1
Total	33,284	78.9	2,203	5.2	221	0.5

Data from MOH budget office records.

Note: Chiclayo is Lambayeque-Amazonas region.

Food		Maintenance		Other		Totals	
Total	%	Total	%	Total	%	Total	%
45	2.8	56	3.5	161	10.2	1,583	100.0
29	2.2	25	1.9	109	8.1	1,338	100.0
24	3.8	22	3.4	46	7.2	638	100.0
48	2.3	53	2.5	245	11.6	2,115	100.0
40	2.6	51	3.3	117	7.5	1,563	100.0
1,027	5.1	798	3.9	1,031	5.1	20,207	100.0
58	3.5	46	2.8	156	9.4	1,665	100.0
82	3.6	71	3.1	278	12.1	2,305	100.0
45	4.3	35	3.3	130	12.3	1,058	100.0
29	2.2	34	2.6	64	4.9	1,315	100.0
74	3.7	56	2.8	214	10.7	2,001	100.0
19	3.1	28	4.6	37	6.1	611	100.0
83	3.2	124	4.8	278	10.8	2,573	100.0
46	3.5	74	5.6	119	9.0	1,320	100.0
26	2.6	37	3.7	108	10.7	1,008	100.0
24	2.7	20	2.3	149	17.0	879	100.0
1,699	4.0	1,530	3.6	3,242	7.7	42,179	100.0

TABLE 8.14

Distribution of MOH Resources
in Relation to Population by Health Region, 1984
(in absolute terms and in percentages)

			MOH RESOURCES					
	Population share		Financial share		Hosp. bed share		HCP share	
Health Regions	Total	%	Total	%	Total	%	Total	%
Piura	1,746,713	9.3	19,783	3.8	496	3.1	154	6.5
Chiclayo	1,375,512	7.3	16,723	3.2	455	2.8	156	6.5
Cajamarca	865,449	4.6	7,982	1.5	131	0.8	88	3.7
Trujillo	1,052,512	5.6	26,431	5.0	439	2.7	120	5.0
Huaraz	929,472	4.9	19,558	3.7	575	3.6	113	4.7
Lima/Callao	5,289,483	28.1	252,582	47.9	8,060	49.8	312	13.1
Ica	697,230	3.7	20,812	3.9	737	4.6	127	5.3
Arequipa	808,600	4.3	28,810	5.5	1,146	7.1	108	4.5
Tacna	280,400	1.5	13,219	2.5	447	2.8	58	2.4
Puno	946,700	5.0	16,435	3.1	407	2.5	130	5.5
Cusco	1,232,807	6.5	25,012	4.7	1,075	6.6	226	9.5
Ayacucho	463,275	2.5	7,633	1.4	251	1.6	68	2.9
Huancayo	1,325,097	7.0	32,164	6.1	878	5.4	279	11.7
Huanuco	880,279	4.7	16,507	3.1	571	3.5	164	6.9
Moyobamba	371,500	2.0	12,599	2.4	216	1.3	147	6.2
Iquitos	559,800	3.0	10,990	2.1	299	1.8	134	5.6
Total	18,824,829	100.0	527,240	100.0	16,183	100.0	2,384	100.0

Data from MOH budget office records.

Note: Chiclayo is Lambayeque-Amazonas region.
Financial share is actual expenditures in millions of current soles.
HCP refers to the combined total of public health centers and posts.

TABLE 8.15

Major Sources of Foreign Aid, 1978 - 87
(in millions of U.S. dollars)

Source	Amount	Implementation	Terms	Objectives
Pan American Health Organization	1.100	1978 - 84	Grant	Maternal and child health care
World Bank	33.500	1983 - 88	Loan	Primary health care expansion
Interamerican Development Bank	0.675	1982 - 84	Grant	Health care training
US Agency for International Development	5.800 1.350	1979 - 85	Loan Grant	Primary health care expansion
US Agency for International Development	4.000 6.900	1981 - 86	Loan Grant	Primary health care expansion and family planning
US Agency for International Development	10.000 1.000	1980 - 87	Loan Grant	Potable water and basic sanitation for villages
German Technical Assistance Program	4.000 1.400	1980 - 85	Loan Grant	Primary health care expansion and hospital renovation
Subtotal	57.300 12.325		Loan Grant	
Total	69.625			

Source: Westinghouse 1985.

9

Medical Care Under Social Security: Coverage, Costs, and Financing

Carmelo Mesa-Lago

This chapter analyzes the coverage, costs and financing of the medical care program of the Peruvian Institute of Social Security (IPSS) in the context of Peru's recent economic recession, which has substantially reduced the institute's revenue base. IPSS spends more on health care annually than the Ministry of Health does (see Chapters 1 and 8), but covers only about half as many people at over twice the cost *per capita*. Moreover, until 1984 coverage applied primarily to adult workers, with only limited health services available to their spouses and infants.

The IPSS medical care program began to operate at a deficit even before the Peruvian economy slid into recession, and continued to do so through 1983. Dramatically deteriorating real wages and widespread non-collection of contributions—especially the government's failure to pay its own employer contributions—began to erode IPSS revenues in the late 1970s, while high administrative and personnel costs, inefficient hospital services, and expensive outside contracting caused increased expenditures. Between 1977 and 1983, medical program spending climbed from 47 to 62 percent of total IPSS expenditures (Table 9.1), and by 1983, despite a pattern of regular IPSS borrowing from its own pension and disability programs to cover the medical care program's deficits, the program had virtually exhausted its contingency reserve.

In its last two years in office, the government of President Fernando Belaunde Terry attempted to address the institute's problems. In 1983, the government began paying its employer contributions, at the same time prohibiting further transfers to the medical care program from other IPSS funds and allowing more enlightened and profitable investment policies for the medical program's reserve funds. In 1984, the government enacted a 1.5 percent increase in contribution rates, but also increased sick pay benefits and extended IPSS medical care coverage to children up to the age of fourteen.

With President Alan Garcia's assumption of the presidency of Peru in July of 1985, the new IPSS administration adopted measures to discourage evasion of contributions and payment delays and to improve operating efficiency. Under the direction of Dr. Jose Barsallo Burga, a key APRA party leader, IPSS was in a favorable political position to lower costs, expand coverage, and increase the efficiency of its medical care program, and in 1985 the program produced a surplus for the first time in ten years. Without substantial improvements in operation and efficiency, however, it is doubtful that the measures taken so far will be sufficient to restore IPSS to a stable financial balance, reduce its operating costs, and improve the accessibility and quality of its medical care program.

Benefits and Coverage

Medical Care Benefits

Under the IPSS medical care program, contributors (salaried workers, the self-employed, and pensioners) are entitled to outpatient medical care, hospitalization, dentistry, certain basic medicines, rehabilitation services, prostheses, and orthopedic aids, as well as sick pay and a funeral allowance. In addition, female enrollees are entitled to paid maternity leave plus an infant nutritional subsidy. Blue-collar workers are covered for occupational accidents and diseases. Spouses of the insured are entitled only to maternity care. Until recently, children under 1 year old received limited health services, such as vaccinations and preventive care; older children were not entitled to any services. Since 1985, children through age 14 have been entitled to receive preventive and ambulatory care and medicines, but no hospitalization. White-collar employees can choose between the services offered by IPSS facilities and contracted public or private services. If the latter are chosen, the insured pays for the service and claims a refund from IPSS according to a pre-determined allowance.

The actual benefits conferred by IPSS fall far short of enrollees' legal entitlements. For example, to qualify their children up to age 14 for the recently extended coverage, insured parents must register them. By the end of 1985 (the first year of expanded coverage), only 40,000 to 60,000 dependent children (about 1.7 to 3.6 percent of the total) had been registered. More generally, stipulated services are not always available to the insured. Medicines are very scarce, sick pay takes two months to process, the infant nutrition subsidy is minimal, and prostheses and orthopedic aids are rarely supplied (CBI 1984; Córdova Cossio 1985). Yet despite this lack of basic services, the law provides for an extravagant benefit that has been afforded to a small number of the insured: treatment abroad when it is not available in Peru.

Estimates of Coverage

Peru's largely unified social security system, created by the merging of several funds in 1973, is legally mandated to cover all salaried workers in the public and private sectors, as well as members of cooperatives and parastatal enterprises (1). The 1984 statute that extended coverage to children of the insured up to the age of fourteen entitled them to preventive health services, ambulatory care, and medicines. Wives of enrollees continue to receive only maternity care. All those receiving IPSS pensions are now fully covered, and the self-employed may join IPSS through voluntary affiliation. There are thus five groups of IPSS beneficiaries, two of them economically active (salaried workers and the self-employed) and three economically inactive (spouses, children to age 14, and pensioners). Although pensioners nominally contribute to IPSS, the two economically active groups constitute the main revenue base of the medical care program. Rough IPSS estimates presented in Table 9.2 indicate an increase in mandated coverage from 15 percent in 1975 to almost 19 percent in 1985.

Effective coverage under the medical care program may well be lower than the 18.6 percent shown in Table 9.2. To begin with, the institute's statistics are deficient. Although a unified registry of social security coverage was legally mandated in 1973 and designed five years later, it has never been implemented. A 1981 census of insured persons proved defective and has never been published. Another national survey of the insured was conducted in 1984, but the sample was skewed toward the larger enterprises and white-collar workers. Since legal marriages and small families are more common among white-collar workers the survey overestimated the number of married insured and underestimated the number of dependent children (2).

Before 1979, IPSS categorized the insured only as blue-collar or white-collar workers. Since 1979, only those actually contributing—not their dependents—have been counted, and the published data do not identify these contributors as salaried, self-employed, or pensioners. The figures for spouses and children are usually estimated by applying fixed ratios to the insured population. Only in 1984 was the first attempt made to provide separate figures for the five categories of insured (IPSS 1984b), and the effort was not sustained in a statistical synopsis published by IPSS in 1985, which reverted to the original blue-collar/white-collar classification and an aggregate figure for all contributors (IPSS 1985a, Table 1.3).

The flaws in the coverage statistics became apparent in a 1984 IPSS actuarial study. In order to calculate the number of economically active insured (salaried plus self-employed), this study tried several different methods. Ultimately, projections from urban employment figures from the 1981 census and from the number of IPSS identification cards were rejected in favor of a combination of the 1984 survey data on the number of insured with statistics on social security contributors. This resulted in a figure of 2.4 million insured, a number close to the one in Table 9.2. However, the figures on dependents remain uncertain and controversial. In estimating the potential number of children between 1-14 to be covered by IPSS, the actuarial study rejected the proportion of the total population in that age group in the 1981 census as a basis for its figures, and instead used IPSS' usual procedure, projecting a fixed ratio of 1.19 children for each insured male. The resulting estimate—2.3 million children (vs. 2.5 million for the other method)—has been questioned by the new IPSS president, who cited a 30 percent lower estimate of 1.65 million late in 1985 (Barsallo 1985, Table 1).

Even if accurate, these coverage statistics do not suggest the number of persons actually qualifying for IPSS medical services, as defined by possession of a medical care program identification card. The 1984 National Household Survey on Health and Nutrition (ENNSA 1984) disclosed that 70 percent of those nominally covered by IPSS had no identification card, and 3 percent held cards that were no longer valid. Only 27 percent held valid cards and were thus guaranteed access to services. This suggests that IPSS statistics on nominal coverage substantially overstate the access of the insured to medical services. As if to confirm this, in late 1985 IPSS published an estimate of the "real" coverage: 15.3 percent of the total 1985 population (not 18.6 percent, as in Table 9.2). Unfortunately, IPSS neither explained the term "real" nor the methods used for its estimate (Barsallo 1985, Table 2). A cautious observer might reasonably conclude that IPSS medical care program coverage is substantially lower than the estimated total: of the 18.6 percent of the population for whom coverage is legally mandated, perhaps three-fourths have paid their contributions and are actually covered, and of those three-fourths not all have access to the services to which they are entitled.

The new IPSS administration has given priority to three important measures which, if implemented, could generate accurate coverage information. One of these—initiating and maintaining a unified registration record—has been awaiting implementation since it was first suggested in 1973. The second—updating individual records of the insured and their employers—is equally necessary. Computerization makes practicable the third—developing an integrated database for the medical care program. To be effective, this database should compile statistics (age, sex, salary or wage, economic activity, employer, and residence) for each IPSS category of insured, and specify whether or not a spouse may have direct entitlement as an employee so as to avoid double counting. Without the orderly compilation of reliable information, the extent of IPSS population coverage will remain uncertain.

Inequalities in Coverage

Although the differences in benefits for blue- and white-collar workers were reduced and coverage extended to domestic servants and self-employed workers in the 1970s, significant differences in IPSS coverage still remain between age groups, geographical areas, economic sectors, and occupational categories. As of 1985, IPSS primarily covered middle-income urban workers in the more developed departments of Peru. Coverage is relatively high among salaried employees in manufacturing, public utilities, transportation, and financial services, while the self-employed and agricultural workers are still largely excluded.

An estimate of IPSS coverage by age group in 1985 is shown in Table 9.3. It is evident that IPSS has concentrated its medical care coverage on the economically active and pensioners, while dependent children have had minimal coverage. The 1984 expansion of coverage to children up to the age of 14 was intended to repair this glaring disparity, but since very few in the newly-entitled age group had actually attained entitlement to benefits by 1985, the figures for that year were not significantly affected by this legislation.

Coverage by department is also very unequal (Table 9.4). In 1981, Lima had the greatest coverage at 27 percent (almost twice the national average), followed by adjacent Callao, the country's main port, with 25 percent. The strikingly heavy concentration of IPSS medical care resources in the Lima metropolitan region is illustrated in Table 9.5. With 31 percent of the country's population, this region contains 58 percent of all Peruvians insured under IPSS. It accounts for 64 percent of the program's total expenditures, and between 50 and 70 percent of all resources and services—although these resources are very inefficiently utilized. Ica, Tacna, and Arequipa—the country's other main urban centers—were also better covered than the national average.

In contrast, the departments with the least coverage (3-4 percent) were Amazonas, Apurimac, Ayacucho, Cajamarca, Huancavelica, and Puno, where the main economic activities are agricultural and where the indigenous Indian populations suffer the worst living conditions in the country (INE 1983a; BCR 1984). Geographic differences in coverage remained virtually unchanged from 1961 to 1981 (Mesa-Lago 1979:136-141).

IPSS medical care coverage by economic sector is more difficult to assess. IPSS has never attempted a sectorial classification of the insured, a gap that Table 9.6 attempts to fill using ENSSA (1984) data on occupation by economic sector together with IPSS data on card-holders. The sectors with the highest coverage are utilities, financial services and insurance, mining, transportation, and manufacturing, while agriculture, trade, and construction are only minimally covered. Underlying these disparities is the fundamental inequality between the formal and informal sectors of the economy (see Chapter 3).

Census data suggest that in 1981 the formal sector accounted for only about 40 percent of the Peruvian labor force. Comparing IPSS nominal coverage data for that year with these census data (Table 9.7) suggests that 90 percent of those employed in the formal sector were legally covered—*i.e.*, they were entitled to benefits under the medical care program, and their employers were legally required to belong to IPSS and to transmit employer and employee contributions to the medical care fund. The same table shows that IPSS enrollment among the self-employed was only about 2 percent, and the unemployed were virtually excluded from coverage. These figures, together with the ENNSA data, imply that there is still a sizable number of formal sector workers—legally covered, according to Table 9.7—who lack the IPSS identification card required for access to medical benefits; still, this sector of the economy (except for dependents) is largely covered by the program. In effect, the relatively small share of the labor force encompassed by the formal sector (the sector most amenable to an orderly and supervisable system of employer/employee contributions) constitutes a serious obstacle to further extension of coverage under the established financing procedure (ECLA 1985).

Projected Coverage Extensions

The preceding analysis suggests that the most pressing needs and greatest opportunities for broader social security coverage lie in the expansion of benefits for current enrollees' dependents and in the extension of the program into the informal sector of the economy. As of late 1985, IPSS was planning to extend full coverage to spouses and children under age 18, and to broaden coverage in the informal urban sectors and in agriculture (IPSS 1985b). Of these intentions, the most readily implementable is the expansion of coverage for dependents, since the program already provides some services for spouses and children. Coverage for some marginal urban workers (*e.g.*, peddlers employed by concessionaires), participants in the government's massive employment creation program (100,000 in 1985 and approximately 200,000 to 300,000 in 1986), and their dependents will be far more difficult to implement. Not only do these workers generally have low and unstable earnings, but (like the self-employed) they are difficult to identify and reach.

Covering the rural sector will be even more difficult, since most peasants and their families are widely dispersed, have very low incomes, and lack the employer's portion of the social security contribution. Moreover, even if coverage for these workers were legally implemented, actual benefits would be severely limited by the lack of health services infrastructure in rural areas (see Chapter 5). The impediments to the rural expansion of IPSS are illustrated by the fate of a 1966 pilot project for rural social security (Seguro Social Campesino) launched in three communities in Junin, chosen for their relatively advanced socioeconomic and political development. The project provided health education, sanitary measures, maternal and child care, and general medical services through health posts that were amply staffed with a physician and five assistants each. Intended for the beneficiaries of agrarian reform in Indian communities and cooperatives who had contributed land and labor to build the health posts and who paid a nominal fee, the project failed because of high costs, inadequate government financing, and wavering community support (IPSS 1983) (3).

IPSS Medical Care Program Operating Costs

From 1975 to 1983, IPSS medical services expenditures increased from 40 to 62 percent of total IPSS expenditures (Table 9.1). The extension of coverage to the 1-14 age group in 1984, according to IPSS estimates, will again increase its medical care expenditures by 18 percent. It is doubtful, however, that the estimated addition of 2.3 million insured (an increase in mandated population coverage from 18 to 30 percent, or a 65 percent increase over the population covered in 1984) can be accomplished—even if the marginal cost of child coverage were kept low by limiting services to preventive and ambulatory care and basic medicines—due to the program's current hospital-centered service structure.

Advisors of the International Labor Organization questioned the feasibility of meeting the new expenditures of this expanded coverage and increased sick pay, and at the same time reducing the system's accumulated financial deficit, through the 1.5 percent contribution rate increase in 1984 (ILO 1984). This skepticism appears entirely justified in view of the remaining persistent causes of the IPSS medical program's high costs in personnel, supplies, and contracted services.

IPSS salaries and fringe benefits increased from 38.5 percent of total operating costs in 1982 to 50.3 percent in 1985. All other costs have proportionately decreased except medical supplies, which showed a slight increase in 1985 (Table 9.8). We lack information on the number of employees in the medical program, but Table 9.9 shows the total number of IPSS employees, in all programs, per 1,000 insured. Between 1975 and 1984, there was a 32 percent increase in the number of IPSS employees, while the number of insured increased by 58 percent. Despite this overall drop in the ratio of employees to insured, however, personnel costs as a percentage of total expenditures continued to climb. In 1984, a Peruvian congressional commission identified several glaring reasons for these soaring costs. Not only were IPSS employees inadequately skilled and personnel control and supervision inefficient, but many employees received salaries without working. In addition, the commission cited problems of labor discipline and union interference in the hiring of IPSS personnel (CBI 1984).

In 1983, there were 20,429 employees in the IPSS medical care program, representing 67 percent of all IPSS employees. Although physicians constitute a sixth of this number at most, they account for a major share of IPSS wage costs. A powerful association and frequent strikes have positioned IPSS doctors among those Peruvians affected least by the decline in real wages in recent years. For IPSS employees of all kinds, personnel recruitment and retention seem to be independent of enrollees' medical needs or the economic viability of the system. In 1976-80, for example, the number of medical personnel at the Hospital Rebagliati, one of the most important in Peru, increased by 50 percent even as the number of daily consultations dropped by 30 percent and hospital income declined by 20 percent (ECLA 1985).

Another expensive component of the program has been its purchase of medical services. Since IPSS does not have facilities in all locations in which it has beneficiaries, and since it sometimes lacks the capacity to provide specialized services, it contracts for these services with the Ministry of Health or with private clinics. Contracted services could conceivably be a lower-cost alternative to the expansion of direct care by IPSS, but they have proved otherwise. Reimbursement for private sector care is determined arbitrarily; there are no reliable estimates of average IPSS medical care costs that could be used to set or compare private sector rates. These rates are also raised every six months according to the inflation rate. Because contracts typically do not specify the medical care to be provided, and neither inspections nor evaluations of the services contracted are required, private clinics frequently get by with inadequate facilities, insufficient and unqualified personnel, and too many patients per office hour (CBI 1984; IPSS 1984a).

The most extravagant medical care program expenditures for contracted services have probably been payments for medical care abroad. From 1978 to 1982, 326 beneficiaries were treated in the US, Canada, the UK, and Spain at a total cost of US $7.25 million. In 1982 alone, 131 insured benefitted from this service at a cost of US $5 million—a figure equivalent to 1.6 percent of total IPSS medical care expenditures for that year. The average cost of this benefit was US $38,168 per beneficiary (IPSS 1984a:32-34.)

In the last few years, IPSS has begun to reduce its dependence on contracted services. The use of these services for outpatient consultations, ambulatory care, and dentistry has declined rapidly from its 1982 peak, as IPSS has expanded its own polyclinics. In 1985, except for the chronically ill, contracted private services were required only outside of Lima. However, for the considerable number of people involved, the cost management problems noted above persist.

In contrast to contracted services, private sector services available to white-collar enrollees have not incurred high costs for IPSS. Because the reimbursement rate has not been readjusted since 1980, the insured absorbs most of the cost of private services. Moreover, considerable time elapses between the application for reimbursement and its payment, and inflation thus reduces its real worth.

Medical Care Financing

Social Security Contributions

The financing of the Peruvian social security program has been highly inefficient and inequitable over the past decade. Between 1975-1984, 93 percent of the revenue of the IPSS medical care program came from wage-based social security contributions, with the balance financed through internal borrowing from other IPSS funds. At the end of 1984, the combined employers' and employees' contribution rate, which had been equivalent to 7.5 percent of employees' pay since the end of 1979, was increased to nine percent. Table 9.10 shows that (within established minimum and maximum limits) salaried and wage-earning employees pay three percent of their total earnings, and employers pay twice that amount. The self-employed and other optionally insured pay nine percent of their earned incomes. Pensioners pay four percent of their pensions, and the pension fund contributes an additional five percent.

The financing system favors higher-income workers over those with lower earnings. Beside the regressive salary ceiling effect noted above (5), the method of determining the contribution ceiling is inequitable. Until the beginning of 1983, the minimum wage of Lima (where about two-thirds of total IPSS medical care program revenue is collected) was the reference point for the national minimum and maximum levels. Since 1983, a standard national "reference unit" has been used, which periodically adjusts the minimum wage to inflation.

Because this adjustment has lagged behind the rapid increase in the cost of living in Peru, the real maximum wage has been substantially reduced: in July of 1985 it was only 52 percent of the July 1981 level, at constant 1979 prices (INE 1985). Thus, although the nominal contribution maximum has gradually increased, the real ceiling has been reduced. This has worsened the regressivity of the established ceiling, because lower-income workers pay a higher proportion of their wages in social security tax than do higher-income workers. This inequity is redressed to some extent by the effect of the established minimum wage, since the contribution for an employee whose salary falls below that minimum is fully paid by the employer.

Government Debt

At the end of 1985, the accumulated debt owed to IPSS by the public and private sectors was conservatively estimated at about US$ 420 million, equivalent to one and a half times the medical care program's annual operating expenditures during the 1980s. Nearly two-thirds of this debt is owed by the public sector (Table 9.11). The government has not only regularly failed to pay its social security contribution as employer; it has also neglected to transfer contributions collected from its employees to IPSS. Nor has the government paid a constitutionally-mandated equivalent of an additional one percent contribution to extend IPSS coverage to the poor before this stipulation was eliminated in the early 1980s. Yet despite the state's debt, IPSS has continued to provide health services to the insured in the public sector, aggravating the medical care program's deficit. Thus, in effect, revenue from private sector contributions has subsidized coverage of public sector employees. Table 9.11 shows the total debt of the public sector to all IPSS programs for the period 1969-1985. Since preliminary IPSS estimates for 1983 showed even greater debts than those reflected in this table (CBI 1984; ECLA 1985), it is safe to say that the debt estimates in the table are conservative.

The real magnitude of the government's debt to IPSS is even greater when one assesses the impact of Peruvian currency devaluation, by calculating the debt in dollars at the official exchange rate when it was incurred and again at the official 1985 rate. Table 9.11 estimates the accumulated loss to IPSS as a result of the devaluation of the *sol* at US $194 million. Had the estimates been made on a yearly basis instead of in periods of 10 to 15 years, the figures would reveal an even greater revenue loss by IPSS.

In 1983 the government attempted to redress its IPSS debt, but so far the result has fallen short of success. In that year it paid 80 percent of its annual contribution as employer, including wage deductions for the insured, and it has continued partial payment since then. The government (including public enterprises) also acknowledged a debt to IPSS of 80 billion *soles* through 1982, and decided to pay this debt with bonds at 56 percent interest. However, since banks then paid 60 percent interest and the inflation rate was 125 percent, the yield of these state bonds was negative. Of course the payment of anything less than the full employer contribution itself contributes to the ongoing accumulation of debt.

At the end of 1985, IPSS accepted an agreement by which the central government contracted to pay off 10 percent of its accumulated debt with new Argentine equipment for 21 hospitals, preferring this type of payment to more of the bonds which had proven so unrewarding (6). Nevertheless, the remaining central government debt continues to devalue with continuing inflation.

Of the remaining public sector debts shown in Table 9.11, the debts of local governments and cooperatives are practically irrecoverable; the overall budget deficits of municipal administrations in Peru are so great that some have stopped paying their employees, and accumulated debts have caused many cooperatives to disband. Public enterprises, such as Pesca Peru, Banco Popular, and the Empresa Nacional de Transporte Urbano, are in a better position to pay their debts, but they still remain substantially in default (7).

Private Sector Evasion and Fines

In similar fashion, private employers have increasingly evaded social security contributions during the 1980s. Moderate estimates for 1985 show that 65 percent of employers either completely evaded their contributions or paid less than the amount required by law, so that 35-40 percent of mandated contributions remained uncollected. The employers' accumulated debt (including their employees' contributions) rose to 437 billion *soles* by mid-1985, or about two thirds the level of the public sector debt. Since these figures take into account only known evaders, however, they significantly underestimate the real private sector debt (8).

One of the main reasons for evasion by employers is IPSS's lack of an employer registry and individual employee accounts. Establishing these is a high-priority objective of the new IPSS administration. From 1968 to 1974, IPSS maintained monthly control of employers' contributions, but this system was discontinued in 1975. It has been extremely difficult since then to construct individual accounts for employers, and impossible to track the individual accounts of the insured (Córdova Cossio 1985). As in the public sector, spiraling inflation also encourages payment delays. Other causes of evasion reported by the congressional commission investigating this problem are a deficient supervision system, illegal agreements between inspectors and debtors, chaotic and often corrupt legal proceedings to collect outstanding debts, and low initiative and efficiency of IPSS lawyers (CBI 1984).

On six occasions between 1975 to 1983, renegotiated payment arrangements were granted to employers in default, but lack of control made them ineffective. Starting in 1984, IPSS took additional steps to address the problem. A moratorium on penalties and interest was declared, allowing up to five years for debt payments, and computerization of accounts has made more efficient control possible. Recognizing that these measures will not necessarily cause those in default to pay, the administration has also refused to provide health services to insured workers whose employers still owe contributions, forcing these employers to negotiate payment agreements with IPSS.

Under PROSIR, a program for social security registration and tax collection, the previous IPSS administration initiated a more ambitious campaign against evasion and default by creating a unified registration record for employers and employees, maintaining up-to-date accounts for both groups and carrying out efficient inspections of employers' records and automatic coercive actions against debtors (9). Employing an updated version of a program used initially from 1967 to 1974 and again from 1978 to 1979, PROSIR planned to institute a national census of employers and employees and national registration prior to its full commencement. Thereafter, each month, IPSS would issue forms on which employers must record payroll changes. Upon receipt of these statements, IPSS would bill employers, who would have to pay the full amount owed at a bank. Receipts for these transactions would be sent to IPSS, which would issue cards entitling insured employees to social security services. All contributions would be registered in the individual accounts of both employers and employees.

If successfully implemented, this new system could provide more prompt and continuous coverage, eliminating the current one-month processing lag between the employer's payment and the issuance of the card entitling the employee to medical services for three months. PROSIR also planned to invoke more stringent sanctions against delinquent employers. An employer who retained the social security contribution of an insured worker instead of transferring it to IPSS would be subject to a prison sentence. If an employer were in default, IPSS would institute collection procedures that might include seizure of property. IPSS would also impose a monthly eight percent interest charge on outstanding debt the first month, doubling the charge in each succeeding month the debt remained unpaid. Although its procedures are cumbersome and the sequence of transactions could be simplified, this new system offers the promise of substantial improvement. A three-year experimental run of PROSIR has produced satisfactory results.

Investments

In the past, the real return on IPSS investments of disability and especially of pension funds has been negative, as Table 9.12 illustrates. In 1981, 31.4 percent of IPSS investments were in construction, mainly of facilities for the medical care program. In 1983, the second largest IPSS investment (21.8 percent) was in inter-program loans, particularly from the other two funds to the medical care program (IPSS 1984d). Because their basic objective is to maintain a contingency reserve to correct temporary imbalances, the investments of the medical care program itself are small. It is not possible to analyze investments of the three IPSS funds or their respective returns separately, since available data lump together all investments and interest accumulated at the end of each year. These pooled data indicate a negative real rate of return on investments until 1984, followed by a dramatic shift to a positive rate of return by mid-1985, when investments were transferred from domestic bank deposits and bonds to bank certificates denominated in foreign currency. This change seems to have been made at the recommendation of the congressional commission in response to the loss in real value of deposits at the Banco de la Nacion (CBI 1984:30, 47; IPSS n.d.).

Financial Equilibrium

Incomplete documentation and inadequate accounting procedures make IPSS accounting balances from 1973 to 1980 unreliable, but they do show that IPSS generated an annual surplus in 1975-84, although this surplus declined from 18.6 percent of total income to 10.3 percent during this time. However, according to the balance sheet this surplus was produced consistently by the pension fund; the medical care fund shows a deficit from 1977 through 1984. Analysis of this deficit is complicated by different sets of revenue and expenditure data, a situation that Table 9.13 attempts to rectify. It includes all medical care revenues and expenditures (current and capital). Revenues include transfers from other programs—pension fund and occupational risks (disability)—and expenditures include the costs of these transfers. The sole exclusion is the indeterminable portion of central administration expenditures attributable to the medical care program; hence expenditures are somewhat underestimated, and the medical fund deficit is actually higher than the table indicates.

For 1975-1984, the cumulative deficit of the medical care program was US $181 million. Between 1977-1982, this deficit increased almost continuously; the one exception to this pattern, the shrinking deficit in 1980, was the result of an increase in contribution rates and in the salary ceiling at the end of 1979.

After reaching its peak in 1982, the deficit declined to a point at which, in 1985, a surplus was achieved for the first time in a decade. Both the 1983-84 deficit reductions and the 1985 surplus were probably the result of more regular employer payments by the government, as well as a gradual reduction of the costs of contracted services and other measures to control expenditures. The change from deficit to surplus in 1985 was also the result of the 1984 increases in contribution rates and salary ceiling, and further actions taken to control expenditures.

Table 9.13 also shows the dramatic erosion of revenues suffered by the medical care program as the result of inflation. Real revenue in 1978 was half that of 1975, and—after increasing in 1981—fell again in 1982-84. Despite the slight recovery of 1985, real revenues for that year were 21 percent below those of 1975 and 45 percent below those of 1981. On the income side, the erosion of the real value of wages and the aggravation of the central government debt are the principal causes of the deficit.

IPSS has traditionally covered its medical care program deficits by borrowing from its pension and disability programs. In 1983 these loans constituted about one fifth of IPSS's total investments. Although further loans of this kind were prohibited in that same year, by July of 1985 the indebtedness of the medical care program to the pension fund still amounted to 173 billion *soles* (10). This figure does not include the pension program's tacit subsidy of the medical care program by assuming most of their common administrative services expenses.

Summary and Conclusions

IPSS devotes substantial resources to medical care, but these resources are unevenly distributed demographically, geographically, and sectorially, and are administered inefficiently. The medical attention provided by these resources is relatively costly, yet some segments of the Peruvian population—most notably the dependent children of workers covered by IPSS—are insufficiently covered. Moreover, the actual benefits delivered under IPSS often fall far short of enrollees' legal entitlements.

In 1985, after the long-overdue adoption of measures to improve its operating efficiency, discourage the evasion of contributions, and speed up its payments, the IPSS medical care program produced a surplus for the first time in ten years. It is doubtful, however, that the measures implemented so far will be sufficient to restore IPSS to a stable financial balance, reduce its operating costs, and improve the accessibility and quality of its medical care program. The policies already implemented or under consideration by the new IPSS administration should therefore be augmented by some of the following measures.

To enhance its financial stability, IPSS might consider eliminating the salary ceiling; instituting progressive contribution rates based on earned income; lobbying for legislation requiring that the government as employer include in its budgets the funds needed to pay its IPSS contributions; taking legal action against employers in default; imposing increased fines on delinquents; proposing legislation allowing contingency fund investments to be made at money market rates of return; and implementing forms of financing other than payroll deductions, so that coverage could be extended to the informal sector and rural population.

To increase the scope of its coverage, IPSS must work toward greater efficiency in administering its medical care program resources. The institute should consider reapportioning these resources, both geographically and sectorially, in favor of the highest-risk populations, with emphasis on rural or urban-marginal primary health care facilities rather than expensive urban hospitals. More specifically, the process through which those who are entitled to medical care—especially newly-entitled children aged 1-14—obtain valid identification cards should be simplified.

In order for IPSS to reduce its operating costs, it must first develop an integrated, computerized database for the medical care program. Other measures that could result in improved cost control include more cautious hiring practices, more attentive personnel supervision, and closer evaluation of the high administrative, personnel, and supply costs associated with hospital services. The costs of contracted services could be better controlled if reliable estimates of average medical care costs were used to establish private sector rates, and inspections or evaluations of contracted services were required. Expensive medical treatment abroad should be eliminated.

After a decade of IPSS deterioration, in which the medical care program failed to meet the most urgent needs of IPSS enrollees and their dependents, the policies of the new administration offer considerable hope for the program's improvement and expansion. If that hope is not to be disappointed, fundamental shifts in the direction and emphases of the program—from curative to preventive care, from large urban hospitals to more widely accessible clinics and polyclinics, from insured workers to their dependents, from the formal sector to the rest of the economy—must be accompanied by equally essential administrative measures. Above all, IPSS must follow through on its plans if it is not to continue the tradition of unfulfilled expectations described in this chapter.

Footnotes

1. The system does not cover several groups with independent programs: the armed forces, police, fishermen, jockeys, and employees of such state-owned enterprises as Petroperu and Centromin.

2. Interview with Homero Gutierrez, Assistant Manager of Statistics, IPSS, December 12, 1985.

3. A more ambitious IPSS project is now being designed to strengthen the rural infrastructure.

4. Data provided in staff interview.

5. In taxation discussions, regressivity refers to the declining proportion paid in by beneficiaries as their incomes rise—particularly once a ceiling beyond which beneficiaries are no longer taxed is reached.

6. Interview with Jose Barsallo Burga, Executive President of IPSS, and Angel Saltachin, Planning and Budget manager of IPSS, Lima, Dec. 10, 1985.

7. Interview with Pablo Concha, Office of Registration, Assessment, and Collection, IPSS, Lima, Dec. 12, 1985.

8. Interviews with Carlos Bockos, Central Manager for Registration, Assessment, and Collection, IPSS, and Cesar Zambrano of the same office, Lima, Dec. 11-12, 1985.

9. This section is based on IPSS, "Sistema de Inscripcion y Recaudacion," Lima, June 1985; and "Proyecto SIR PROSIR," Lima, August 1985.

10. Interview with Rosa Lopez, Economic Counselor, Executive Presidency, IPSS, Lima, Dec. 12, 1985.

TABLE 9.1

Proportion of Total IPSS Expenditures Allotted to Medical Care: 1975-1984

Year	Total expenditures	Medical care* expenditures	Medical care expenditures as percentage of total expenditures
	(in billions of Soles)		
1975-76	31.1	12.5	40.2
1977	22.1	10.4	47.0
1978	33.3	16.9	50.8
1979	61.2	33.0	53.9
1980	128.2	67.3	52.5
1981	233.2	144.1	61.8
1982	380.0	235.4	61.9
1983	630.2	389.9	61.8
1984	1,188.2	638.4	53.7

* – Includes monetary and medical–hospital benefits of the Medical Care Program and medical–hospital benefits of the occupational risks program.

Sources: Estimates based on IPSS 1985a and Table 9.13.

TABLE 9.2

Estimated Population Coverage by the Peruvian Social Security Medical Care Program, 1975-1985

(in thousands)

	Contributing Insured				Dependents				
Year	Salaried[a]	Self-employed	Pensioners[b]	Sub-total A	Spouses[c]	Children[d]	Sub-total B	Total A+B	Total Population
1975	1,562	17	146	1,725	—507—		507	2,232	15,161
1980	2,014	39	211	2,264	546	66	612	2,876	17,295
1981	2,093	50	230	2,373	554	68	622	2,995	17,755
1982	2,167	61	243	2,471	572	70	642	3,113	18,226
1983	2,243	74	256	2,573	705	102	807	3,380	18,707
1984	2,321	87	270	2,678	734	105	839	3,517	19,198
1985	2,403	101	283	2,787	765	109	874	3,661	19,698

(in percentages of total population)

1975	10.3	0.1	1.0	11.4	—3.3—		3.3	14.7	100
1980	11.6	0.2	1.2	13.1	3.2	0.4	3.5	16.6	100
1981	11.8	0.3	1.3	13.4	3.1	0.4	3.5	16.9	100
1982	11.9	0.3	1.3	13.6	3.1	0.4	3.5	17.1	100
1983	12.0	0.4	1.4	13.8	3.8	0.5	4.3	18.1	100
1984	12.1	0.5	1.4	13.9	3.8	0.5	4.4	18.3	100
1985	12.2	0.5	1.4	14.1	3.9	0.6	4.4	18.6	100

Notes: a - Includes domestic workers. Excludes independently-covered armed forces, police, fishermen, and jockeys.
b - Includes old age disability-survivor and occupational-risk pensioners in private and public sectors. Excludes pensioners from armed forces, police, fishing and racetracks.
c - Spouses of active and passive insured entitled only to maternity care.
d - Children under one year old entitled to out-patient care. 1984 extension to age 14 not yet widely implemented.

Source: 1983-1985 IPSS estimates, as reported to author; 1975-1982 estimates based on IPSS internal figures.

TABLE 9.3

IPSS Medical Care Coverage Distribution by Age Group: 1985

Age Group	Percent of total population	Percent of IPSS insured	Percent of age group covered[a]
0-14[b]	40.2	3.0	1.4
15-59	54.4[c]	87.2[c]	29.9
60 and over	5.4	9.8	33.8
Total	100.0	100.0	18.6

Notes: a - Number of insured divided by total population in age group.
b - Almost exclusively 0-1 year olds, because of limited implementation of extension to age 14.
c - Includes spouses entitled only to maternity care. Number of spouses estimated at 90% of insured.

Sources: Population, World Bank estimate for 1985; insured, Table 9.2.

TABLE 9.4

IPSS Medical Care Coverage Distribution by Department: 1981

Department	Percent of population covered[a]
Amazonas	3.1
Ancash	9.8
Apurimac	2.5
Arequipa	17.4
Ayacucho	2.8
Cajamarca	2.7
Callao	24.6
Cusco	4.7
Huancavelica	3.7
Huanuco	4.7
Ica	20.5
Junin	9.5
La Libertad	12.0
Lambayeque	15.0
Lima	26.7
Loreto	8.5
Madre de Dios	6.1
Moquegua	13.9
Pasco	13.1
Piura	8.3
Puno	3.7
San Martin	5.0
Tacna	19.6
Tumbes	8.6
Ucayali	7.5
National Average	14.0[b]

Notes: a - Excludes the armed forces.
b - Difference from figure in Table 9.2 (16.9 percent) attributable to different sources.

Sources: INE 1983b; BCR 1984.

TABLE 9.5

Concentration of IPSS Medical Services in Lima: 1983

Lima	% of Peru total
Total Population (Lima-Callao)	31.0
IPSS Insured (Lima-Callao)	57.8
Health Expenditures (Region)	63.5
Hospital Beds	56.0
Clinics	55.0
Doctors	70.0
Nurses and Technicians	68-75
Out-Patient visits	60.6
Surgical interventions	57.0
Hospital expenditures	56.0
Attended births	62.2
Vaccinations	58.0
Laboratory tests	67.0
Dental care	52.0

Sources: IPSS 1984a; IPSS 1984c. Primary data obtained directly from IPSS.

TABLE 9.6

IPSS Medical Care Coverage by Economic Sector: 1984
(In thousands)

Branch	Total survey	Hold IPSS card	Percent of labor force covered*
Agriculture, livestock forestry, and fishing	201.1	11.0	5.5
Mining	9.7	6.6	68.0
Manufacturing	71.6	28.1	39.2
Construction	21.6	7.2	33.6
Utilities	2.6	2.2	83.5
Transport, warehousing and communications	23.6	10.3	43.7
Trade, restaurants and hotels	107.8	20.2	18.7
Financial services, insurance, etc.	13.7	9.3	67.7
Communal, social, and personal services	111.7	54.9	49.1
Not specified	.8	.4	45.6
Total/Average	564.2	150.1	26.6

* - Percentage based on total absolute figures.

Sources: ENNSA 1984.

TABLE 9.7

IPSS Medical Care Coverage Distribution by Occupational Category: 1981

Occupational Category	Labor force (thousands)	Labor force %	Insured (thousands)	Insured %	Percent covered
Salaried[a] (Formal sector)	2,324	40	2,093	98	90.1
Self-employed	2,150	37	50[b]	2	2.3
Unpaid family worker	443[c]	8	0	0	0
Unemployed	392	7	0	0	0
Not specified	461[c]	8	0	0	0
Total Average	5,770	100	2,143	100	37.1

Notes: a - Includes blue and white-collar and domestic workers.
b - Optionally insured.
c - Figures given by the National Statistical Institute adjusted with figures from ILO.

Sources: Civilian Labor Force from INE 1984, adjusted with ILO 1983; insured workers from Table 9.2

TABLE 9.8

Distribution of IPSS Medical Care Expenditures by Budgetary Item: 1981-1985
(in percentages)

Item	1981	1982	1983	1984	1985
Salaries and fees	39.5	38.5	43.5	48.2	50.3
Medical supplies	20.0	20.0	21.8	20.9	24.3
Contracted and free-choice services	20.7	21.9	18.1	18.0	15.0
Monetary benefits	17.1	18.0	16.0	12.8	10.4
Capital goods	2.7	1.6	0.6	0.1	0.0
Total	100.0	100.0	100.0	100.0	100.0

Source: Estimates based on Barsallo 1985.

TABLE 9.9

IPSS Employees and Remuneration: 1975-1984

Year	No. of IPSS employees	No. of insured* (thousands)	IPSS employees per 1,000 insured	Remuneration as percentage of total social security expenditures
1975	21,598	2,232	9.4	21.6 (1975–1976)
1976	22,000	...	...	
1977	23,503	...	...	24.4
1978	23,900	...	...	25.8
1979	24,136	...	...	26.4
1980	26,850	2,876	9.3	25.4
1981	27,151	2,995	9.1	27.3
1982	30,791	3,113	9.9	27.4
1983	30,200	3,380	8.9	30.5
1984	28,604	3,517	8.1	29.6

* - In medical care program.

Sources: Employees and remuneration from IPSS 1985a; insured figures from Table 9.2.

TABLE 9.10

Legally Mandated Contributions to IPSS: 1985

(as percentage of insured's salary or income)

Programs	Employee	Employer	Total	Self-employed	Pensioners
Medical care	3.0	6.0	9.0	9.0	4.0[a]
Pensions	3.0	6.0	9.0	9.0	0
Occupational risk	0	4.0[b]	4.0	0	0
Total	6.0	16.0	22.0[c]	18.0	4.0

Notes: a - Pension program contributes additional 5%.
b - National average; premium varies from 1 to 12.5% according to risk.
c - Within specified minimum and maximum earnings limits.

Source: Current legislation.

TABLE 9.11

Public Sector Debt[a] to IPSS and Its Devaluation: 1969-1985

Sector	Period	Debt in current soles (billions)	Debt in dollars[b] (millions)	Debt in 1985 dollars	Devaluation loss in current dollars (millions)
Central government[c]	1969-79[d]	13.8	59.7	1.4	58.3
	1980-82	23.2	30.6	2.4	28.2
	1983	92.7	52.0	9.8	42.2
	1984	240.9	61.0	25.4	35.6
	1985[e]	272.5	28.7	28.7	0
Sub-total	1969-85	643.1	232.0	67.7	164.3
Public enterprises	1969-84	98.5	25.0	10.4	14.6
Local governments[d]	1969-84	50.0	12.7	5.3	7.4
Parastatal enterprises	1975-81	3.6	8.1	0.4	7.7
Total		795.2	277.8	83.8	194.0

Notes: a - Including delinquency (mora).
b - Based on official exchange rate at end of debt period.
c - Includes central government, central public institutions, national university and CORDES.
d - Metropolitan Lima only.
e - Preliminary estimate.

Source: Estimated from IPS sources provided by the Gerencia Central de Inscripcion, Acotacion y Recaudacion, Grupo Central de Adeudos, December 12, 1985.

TABLE 9.12

Annual Yields on Financial Investments Made by the IPSS Medical Care Program: 1980-1985

Type of Investment	Yields (percent)											
	1980		1981		1982		1983		1984		1985[b]	
	Nominal	Real[a]	Nominal	Real	Nominal	Real	Nominal	Real	Nominal	Real	Nominal	Real
Deposit Certificates	40.5	-20.3	65.9	-6.8	67.4	-5.5	79.6	-45.5	79.6	-31.9	73.7	-92.4
Parastatal bonds and internal debt	6.0	-54.8	6.0	-66.7	6.0	-66.9	6.0	-119.1	6.0	-105.5	6.0	-160.1
Mortgage bonds									19.5	-92.0	19.5	-146.6
Bank Certificates (US dollars)									10.1	10.1[c]	10.3	10.3
Rate of Inflation	60.8		72.7		72.9		125.1		111.5		166.1	

Notes: a - Nominal yield minus inflation rate.
b - Annual forecast, based on September 1985.
c - Average; fluctuated from 9.8% to 10.3%.

Source: Estimates based on IPSS, "Estudio de la situacion financiera del IPSS," Lima, September 1985, and information from Asesoria Economica de la Gerencia de Finanzas, December 12, 1985.

TABLE 9.13

Income and Expenditures of the IPSS Medical Care Program: 1975-1985

Year	Billions of soles at current prices			Billions of soles in 1975 constant prices			Balance (Percent)	Balance[c] (in millions of dollars)
	Income[a]	Expenditures[b]	Balance	Income	Expenditures	Balance		
1975	6.9	5.4	1.5	6.9	5.4	1.5	21.7	34.2
1976	8.4	7.1	1.3	5.8	4.9	0.9	15.5	22.7
1977	9.0	10.4	(1.4)	4.7	5.4	(0.7)	(15.6)	(16.0)
1978	12.9	16.9	(4.0)	3.9	5.1	(1.2)	(31.0)	(24.3)
1979	23.7	33.0	(9.3)	4.3	5.9	(1.7)	(39.2)	(40.2)
1980	63.6	67.3	(3.7)	7.1	7.5	(0.4)	(5.8)	(12.3)
1981	127.9	144.1	(16.2)	8.3	9.4	(1.1)	(12.7)	(36.4)
1982	175.5	235.4	(59.9)	6.6	8.8	(2.2)	(34.1)	(78.9)
1983	349.8	389.9	(40.1)	5.8	6.5	(0.7)	(11.5)	(22.5)
1984	608.3	638.4	(30.1)	4.8	5.0	(0.2)	(4.9)	(7.6)
1985[d]	1,838.6	1,654.3	184.3	5.4	4.9	0.5	10.0	19.4

Notes: a – Includes current and capital income of the Medical Care Program, pension fund contributions for pensioners, and current and capital income transferred from occupational risks funds (excluded 1975–79).

b – Includes operational and capital expenditures but not central administrative costs of the Medical Care Program and Occupational Risks Program (the latter is excluded in 1975–79).

c – Estimates based on annual average offical exchange rate.

d – Preliminary estimates based on figures at the begining of December.

Sources: Estimates based on IPSS 19885a, 1985c and information from the IPSS Planning and Budget Agency, December 12–13, 1985

10

Health Care in Peru: Inferences and Options

Gretchen Gwynne and Dieter K. Zschock

The foregoing chapters lead to a number of important conclusions and policy options, for consideration particularly by the Government of Peru, the country's private health sector leaders, and international donor agencies, but also, more generally, by all those concerned with the pursuit of universal objectives in international health. Any research project of the magnitude of the HSA-Peru could, of course, support many and diverse conclusions—including some that would no doubt be at odds with those reached in this chapter. Likewise, the recommendations we make could be extended, and alternate options offered, depending on how one interprets the project's rich database. The authors who contributed to this book have not sought to provide concrete answers to policy questions so much as to stimulate informed debate on the most important health care issues facing Peru today. Moreover, they encourage decision-makers to consider these issues within the context not only of the Peruvian health sector but also of the economic, social and political environment of Peru in the 1980s.

Findings and Implications

Of Peru's population of 19 million in 1984, approximately 11 million were medically indigent, and thus depended on the Ministry of Health to provide them with health care, including essential medicines. But the Ministry was able to serve only five million of these needy Peruvians, leaving six million without access to modern health care. Eight million others had access to health services that did not have to be supported through the Ministry. Four million of these were entitled to medical care under the Peruvian Social Security Institute and other privileged public sector programs, and an additional four million had financial access to private sector health services.

Despite the government's policy emphasis on primary health care, and possibly some net increase in total financial support for PHC, the Peruvian health sector is not yet organized for the effective prevention of illness and death in Peru. Across all age groups, respiratory ailments, intestinal infections and accidents are the leading causes of illness and death. Neonatal deaths account for close to half of all infant mortality, while immuno-preventive diseases cause the largest share of child mortality. These preventable ailments account for over three-fourths of all expenditures for curative care.

The underlying causes of illness and death in Peru are the country's hazardous environmental conditions and the population's poverty, low educational levels, and high fertility. While the birth and death rates have declined recently and population growth has slowed to 2.5 percent annually, further improvement in the health status of Peruvians will require concurrent improvements in other socioeconomic indicators. This limits the impact that geographically-expanded primary health care coverage can be expected to have.

Encouraging community participation in the determination of health needs and in the organization and delivery of health services is strongly emphasized under the new government's health sector policy. In a country as geographically, economically, and culturally diverse as Peru, however, there can be no uniform, nation-wide approach to encouraging community participation, since communities' varied ethnic and political characteristics, economic conditions, and past experiences with health program development all affect the degree and effectiveness of their participation. Peruvian examples have shown that effective community participation in health care is seldom imposed from the top down; more often, it arises from within a community. Health care activities initiated from outside a community by the MOH or PVOs are thus apt to be less successful than locally-initiated activities. Yet recent attempts to regionalize health services administration have not led to any significant delegation, to regional and community levels, of authority over program orientation and corresponding resource allocation; authority for the Peruvian health sector remains centralized in Lima.

When the Peruvian health sector is viewed as a whole, it is apparent that two-thirds of all hospitals, medical personnel, medicines, and corresponding financial commitments are concentrated in the country's major urban centers, where they are accessible to only one-third of the population. Primary health care facilities are more evenly distributed throughout Peru, but tend to be poorly maintained, inadequately staffed, and seriously lacking in essential medicines.

The Ministry of Health, considering that it accounts for only 27 percent of Peru's total health sector expenditures, is severely overburdened with the responsibility of financing and managing 54 percent of the country's hospital beds and 86 percent of its primary health care facilities. Annually, the Ministry spends approximately US $30 *per capita* on hospital services, but only US $10 *per capita* on primary health care for the five million Peruvians it covers. The country's private voluntary organizations also spend about US $10 *per capita*, but they cover only two million inhabitants. PVO health services, however, are generally more adequately staffed and supplied than MOH services at the primary care level.

Peru's 1982-83 economic recession significantly reduced the Ministry's financial resources, in real terms. So that jobs would be protected, expenditures were sharply reduced in other areas, such as facilities maintenance and essential medicines. (The Ministry's payments for wages and benefits actually increased, in real terms, over this period.) As of 1984, the major determinants of MOH expenditures by health region were hospital costs, rather than more urgently needed primary health care support.

Medical care under the Peruvian Institute of Social Security covers 3.5 million Peruvians (about 18 percent of the population), but IPSS accounts for 33 percent of total health sector expenditures. Wage-based contribution rates have been increased, yet—because of traditionally high costs and the widespread evasion of social security contributions on the part of employers—the IPSS medical care program has operated at a deficit for the past 10 years. The 1982-84 economic recession also sharply reduced IPSS revenues, at the same time that the government mandated an expansion of IPSS coverage to include beneficiaries' children to age 14.

On average, hospital stays in both MOH and IPSS facilities are twice as long in Peru as they are in comparable Latin American countries. Private sector hospitals, which are among the newest facilities available, are underutilized, probably because of their high charges compared to the low user fees charged for inpatient care in public sector hospitals. If the average length of stay at public sector facilities were reduced, Peru would have a surplus of hospital beds, and new construction or even the rehabilitation of a substantial number of older facilities would be unnecessary, except to reduce inequities in the regional distribution of hospitals.

The recent economic recession caused combined public sector health care expenditures (by the MOH, IPSS, and other agencies) to decline from US $595 million in 1981 to US $487 million in 1984. The resulting curtailment of health services by the MOH and IPSS has undermined public confidence in the quality of public sector health care, and increased the demand for private care. Those Peruvians who do consult public sector practitioners prefer hospital-based services over those offered by health centers and posts; the reasons are perceived differences in quality and accessibility.

Throughout the recession, total health sector expenditures remained constant, in relative terms, at 4.5 percent of GDP, but they would have declined even in relative terms were it not for two factors: the absolute increase of close to US $30 million in private health care expenditures, and foreign aid contributions totaling between US $30 and $40 million.

Private health sector expenditures in Peru include direct household and employer payments for medical services, risk-sharing arrangements through private health insurance and other prepayment mechanisms, and expenditures for health care made by cooperatives and private voluntary organizations. During the recent recession, private expenditures through risk-sharing arrangements appear to have increased, while expenditures through cooperatives and PVOs apparently declined. Overall, however, private health care expenditures increased in real terms, from approximately US $218 million to US $245 million over this period. In Lima, over one-third of all ambulatory care visits reported by households are private sector consultations, and in the urban areas of the mountain states this proportion is close to two-thirds.

Private sector prepaid health care arrangements in Peru are apparently confined, thus far, to the Lima/Callao metropolitan area. Their emergence over the past 10 years has largely been a reaction to the declining quality of public sector services—particularly medical care provided by IPSS. There is reason to expect that IPSS services will improve, and that coverage for enrollees' dependents will be further expanded—developments that would tend to reduce the pressure on employers to provide private health care alternatives for their workers. These possibilities, together with unstable employment conditions and the low absolute incomes of a large proportion of the capital area's population, mitigate against the rapid expansion of private sector health care financing alternatives.

Foreign aid disbursements in 1982-84 represented between six and seven percent of total MOH expenditures, with most of this aid earmarked for the Ministry's primary health care program, initiated in 1982. In 1984, foreign aid accounted for about one-third of all MOH primary health care expenditures. Over this same period, the MOH sharply reduced its transfer payments to PVOs in order to meet the financial requirements of its own programs. Thus international donors may unwittingly have encouraged a shift in the composition of Peruvian primary health care expenditures from the private to the public sector, reducing the economic strength of PVOs at the expense of increased MOH spending for primary health care.

Peruvian medical personnel, who in general prefer to work in hospitals rather than in primary care facilities, are concentrated in the major urban areas of the country, where many rural Peruvians cannot gain access to them. The heaviest urban concentration is evident for MOH employees, including not only medical doctors but also PHC workers such as auxiliary nurses; IPSS and private sector practitioners are somewhat more widely scattered, although they, too, are unevenly dispersed in relation to population distribution. One reason for the uneven distribution of health care personnel is that Peruvian medical doctors and registered nurses tend to work near the professional schools from which they graduated, and such schools are largely located in urban settings. To a lesser extent, medical personnel also have a preference for locating near their birthplaces.

Peruvian expenditures for pharmaceuticals totaled US $200 million in 1984, or 27 percent of total health sector expenditures. With most of the 13 million Peruvians covered by modern health services in both the public and private sectors purchasing at least some of their medicines from private pharmacies, private sales—which average US $11 *per capita* annually—constitute nearly three-fourths of all pharmaceutical sales in the country. Meanwhile, government price controls on pharmaceuticals have hampered sales and have contributed to a sharp decline in production in recent years. Subsidiaries of multinational pharmaceutical companies have been most severely affected by worsening market conditions in Peru, causing many of them to discontinue operations. Market shares of wholly-owned domestic manufacturers of pharmaceutical products have increased as a result, but many specialty products, as well as most essential medicines, are now in very short supply.

Recommendations and Policy Options

Under a government that has expressed a strong commitment to improving health care for all Peruvians, and with economic recovery underway, Peruvian health sector leaders and international donors now have an opportunity to make significant progress toward improving the performance of the country's health sector. The research results of the Health Sector Analysis of Peru support a number of specific recommendations and policy options, itemized below, for consideration by Peruvian health sector authorities, both public and private, and by representatives of international donor agencies. These recommendations address matters of immediate priority that should be considered during the current government's term of office.

The Public Health Sector

Leaders of the MOH and IPSS should significantly improve the quality of care offered by their existing services before greatly expanding their health services coverage, since the public sector's financial resources are insufficient for the achievement of both objectives within the time span of the current government's incumbency. Evidence produced by the HSA-Peru suggests that popular confidence in the quality of existing services needs to be improved, particularly at the level of primary health care. Significant expansion of coverage is unlikely to be effective as long as public health services do not have the confidence of the population they are intended to serve.

In particular, the MOH should improve the quality of its primary health services. This will require reallocating some expenditures from hospitals to health centers and posts, which could be accomplished by deactivating a few of the most antiquated MOH hospitals; turning over some MOH hospitals to private sector health care providers (including PVOs); reducing the average length of stay of patients in MOH hospitals; reassigning medical personnel from hospitals to primary health care facilities; improving the maintenance of buildings and equipment at the remaining hospitals and primary health care facilities; and providing all health services with adequate quantities of essential medicines and other important supplies and services.

Maintaining the physical infrastructure of both MOH and IPSS facilities will require a systematic program of simplified surveys—like the one carried out by the HSA-Peru for MOH facilities in Cusco and Cajamarca—to assess the condition of buildings, utility systems, and equipment. There is also a need for a data-processing system on physical infrastructure, utility systems, and equipment, so that administrators can readily assess the overall state of each.

Hospital services provided by the MOH and IPSS should be limited to their respective target populations, and should furthermore be restricted to the provision of essential secondary- and tertiary-level services in direct support of primary health care. Hospital services that are not considered essential should either be left to private sector hospitals or should require significant co-payments from patients. If individuals who are not among the target populations of the MOH or IPSS are to be served in public sector health care facilities—both hospitals and primary health care facilities—they should be charged user fees equivalent to private sector charges.

Public health sector institutions, particularly the MOH and IPSS, need appropriately-designed and efficiently-administered personnel policies, in order to relieve the inequitable distribution of medical personnel. Incentive structures should be devised to reward service at the primary health care level (particularly in currently underserved urban poverty zones, small towns, and outlying rural health posts), so as to reduce the general preference of health care professionals for work in hospital settings. Incentives should include not only adequate remuneration, fringe benefits, and pensions, but also opportunities for professional advancement and the delegation of health care decision-making to lower levels of personnel. Since Peruvian medical doctors and registered nurses tend to work near the professional schools from which they graduated and—to a lesser extent—near their birthplaces, it might be possible to affect the distribution of the country's medical personnel by judicious medical school admissions policies.

Given the proclivity of Peruvians for seeking ambulatory health care in public hospitals rather than health centers or posts, MOH hospitals should reduce the volume of the ambulatory care they provide by strictly limiting access to such care to the medically indigent, if necessary initiating user fees to control access to outpatient services. This effort can succeed, however, only if primary health care facilities are improved and made more accessible—which may require constructing additional health centers and posts in underserved urban areas, including metropolitan Lima.

The MOH budget should be restructured so as to require allocations of adequate funds for facilities maintenance, essential medicines, necessary transportation, and other important recurrent cost items. This means that personnel costs will have to be reduced from their current level of 70 percent to below 60 percent of total expenditures. The most practical way to accomplish such a reduction would be to assign all hospital cost savings, all income from user fees, and any additional funds that may become available to the currently underbudgeted categories, at the same time limiting increases in personnel expenditures to the minimum necessary to maintain adequate working incentives.

Peru's public health sector institutions need a coordinated and equitable program that provides essential medicines, in sufficient quantity, to all their health services, and that strictly limits the distribution of essential medicines to their target populations. The current shortage of essential medicines, as well as the lack of professional and popular confidence in these medicines, must be remedied. This requires that generic medicines must in fact be qualitatively equivalent to brand-name products, differing from them only in packaging and marketing.

In view of the importance of the private sector in the manufacture, distribution, and retail sales of pharmaceutical products in Peru, the MOH should re-examine its current price control policy. While continuing to control prices in order to insure that pharmaceuticals are affordable for the lower middle class (if not for the poor), the government should allow private pharmaceuticals concerns to reap reasonable profits. In addition, the possibility of selling essential medicines through private pharmacies in the form of generic as well a brand-name products should be explored. The government should promote foreign investment in the Peruvian pharmaceuticals industry in such a way that technology transfer is encouraged, and should assist indigenous firms to gradually diversify their production and thus increase their market shares.

The MOH should settle on a single, sustainable, effective approach to the regionalization of health services administration. It needs to decide precisely which administrative functions can be delegated and which ones must be retained at the central level; what reporting requirements are essential and which ones can be eliminated; how impediments to timely financial accounting and the orderly flow of payments can be removed; what form of personnel policy will best stabilize employment conditions without inhibiting upward and geographical mobility; and how MOH responsibilities at the regional and local levels can be made more compatible with the Ministry's policy of encouraging community participation in health care administration and services delivery.

The medical care program of IPSS should be reoriented toward primary health care, and the recent mandate to expand IPSS coverage to covered workers' children—an estimated 2.5 million of them—should be promptly implemented, since covering these children would significantly reduce the pressure on MOH services in urban areas. Current IPSS efforts to reduce the evasion of contributions on the part of employers, together with an agreement by the government as employer to pay its required contributions in full, should make this expansion of coverage possible. IPSS should also implement its intended expansion of coverage in rural areas, under an agreement with rural cooperatives.

IPSS should stabilize its medical care program fiscally, and should cease subsidizing that program with credits from other benefit programs. Since no increase in contribution rates is expected, the collection ratios for contributions must be increased, and operating costs reduced. Medical services should be tailored to the essential care needed by most beneficiaries, based on prevailing patterns of illness; high-cost and non-essential care should be reduced. Wages and benefits for IPSS medical personnel should be contained, and more auxiliary practitioners employed to staff the Institute's new polyclinics (equivalent to MOH primary health care facilities). Finally, IPSS revenues and reserves should be deposited at market rates of interest—not at negative rates, as has been the case in the past.

Together, Peru's public health sector institutions should create an integrated database reflecting the current health status of the Peruvian population, so that both primary health care and hospital services can be oriented toward the leading causes of morbi-mortality. Substantial epidemiological information currently exists, but so far Peru has been unable to make good use of these data—a situation that could be remedied by strengthening the analytical capability of researchers to identify the major determinants of each leading cause of illness and death. Peru's several public and private sector centers for health services research should be supported more strongly and in a manner that encourages coordination and cross-fertilization among them, and the MOH and IPSS should employ a core staff of experienced health planners who would use research findings for specific health services planning. Both researchers and planners will require intensive training in analytical and programming skills before they can make better use of existing databases and assemble improved ones.

The Private Health Sector

Leaders of private institutions in the Peruvian health sector should establish a common forum within which to analyze and debate their role in providing Peruvians with improved and expanded health services coverage at affordable prices. Under the aegis of this private sector forum, the market for hospital and ambulatory care under different cost and price alternatives should be analyzed—an effort likely to demonstrate to the private sector the advantages of expanding financial risk-sharing mechanisms for the populations they serve. Depending on the increase in demand for private hospital care after risk-sharing coverage of the urban middle class has been increased, private sector leaders may find it economically feasible to operate some public hospitals, which the MOH may decide to turn over to them under its own cost reduction plan. Lease arrangements may prove mutually beneficial to both the MOH and private sector interests, providing a new revenue source for the MOH while reducing its expenditures, and giving private sector medical services access to hospital facilities without the need to finance the cost of purchasing them or constructing new facilities.

The Peruvian health insurance industry has seen significant growth in the past 10 years, but is currently facing competition from brokers and employers who are creating self-insurance plans in order to save on health insurance costs. The industry should take this competitive threat as a signal to lower its costs by expanding and becoming more efficient, both in its payments to health care providers and its reimbursements to policy-holders. Further growth would also increase the market power of the industry—especially its ability to contain hospital costs.

Private health care providers who have initiated prepayment plans for individual subscribers should be encouraged to expand their coverage under these plans. There is potential demand among middle- and lower-middle-income Peruvians for such coverage, as long as fees are set at a reasonably low proportion of disposable household income—no more than 3-5 percent, or approximately US $30-50 annually per person. For this prepayment fee, providers should design a package of primary health care and essential hospitalization services that allows them to cover costs and still earn a reasonable profit. Alternatively, such prepaid provider plans should be organized by—or in cooperation with—private voluntary organizations already providing primary health care.

Leaders of urban cooperatives providing health care benefits to their members should reevaluate their programs in light of the expansion by IPSS of coverage for dependent children, and in the face of the emergence of employer- and provider-organized health plans. If cooperatives' health care benefits duplicate services provided for their members under other alternatives, cooperatives should either reduce their benefits or enter into agreements with alternative payment and provider mechanisms to co-finance their members' coverage.

Leaders of rural cooperatives should accept IPSS initiatives to assume responsibility for medical care coverage for their members—if IPSS can guarantee them access to primary health care at polyclinics and, when necessary, referrals to IPSS hospitals. Some increase in rural cooperatives' allocation of financial resources may be necessary for them to obtain medical care coverage under IPSS. An alternative for rural cooperatives might be to contract for health services with private voluntary organizations. In either case the cooperatives, instead of insisting on hospital-based services provided by medical doctors, should recognize the importance of obtaining good primary health care for their members.

Leaders of private voluntary organizations, which have heretofore played a significant role in the private health sector, should reassess this role in light of the virtual elimination of transfer payments by the MOH. Many PVOs have tended to become increasingly dependent on public sector subsidies, including medical personnel paid by the MOH. PVOs should maintain a closely cooperative relationship with the Ministry's primary health care program, but should become administratively and financially independent of the MOH.

By continuing to charge user fees for good quality primary health care, PVOs can cover a substantial part of their operating costs, but—consistent with their origins—they will continue to depend on financial or in-kind support from international and domestic charities and religious organizations. By serving lower-middle-income Peruvians who can afford to pay user fees, PVOs can help the MOH concentrate on serving the medically indigent, often within the same communities. In many cases, PVOs are particularly well suited to working with community leaders toward encouraging community participation. If the Ministry accepts the help of PVOs, these organizations can assist in making the primary health care provided by the MOH more effective within a community.

International Donors

International donor agencies should recognize that, given their own resource constraints, their financial contributions are unlikely to (and probably should not) exceed five percent of total annual health sector expenditures in Peru, and that they therefore cannot expect to exercise strong influence over the country's health policy. Under its past two governments, Peru has been committed to the development of a comprehensive primary health care program, and the current government seems determined to implement an even more ambitious sector-wide primary health care focus. Foreign donors should support this initiative financially, but should accept the Peruvian government's policy orientation rather than imposing alternate models or requirements that may appear to Peruvian health sector authorities as being at odds with their policies.

If international donors were to concentrate most of their aid on the MOH, on the premise that the MOH shares their policy priority to expand primary health care coverage for the medically indigent, then their combined support could account for as much as 20 percent of total MOH expenditures annually over the next three years. In that case, however, donors should be seriously concerned about the Ministry's absorptive capacity and about the likelihood that the MOH would use more foreign aid than domestic financing to expand PHC coverage. If only about half of the international aid for health care were allocated to the MOH, the need for the Ministry to reallocate financial resources and medical personnel from urban hospitals to urban and rural primary health care facilities would be much more pressing, and the likelihood that the MOH could in the future finance the recurrent costs of improved and expanded primary health care services would be increased. In general, donors should assist the MOH to improve existing facilities and programs, rather than encourage the rapid expansion of coverage into rural areas where no services currently exist.

Instead of continuing to concentrate their support on the MOH, international donors should allocate half of their funds for Peru to the IPSS and private sector initiatives, primarily PVOs. In part, the rationale for such a distribution would be to help relieve the Ministry of some of its obligations to finance and manage urban hospitals. Specifically, foreign aid earmarked for IPSS should be used to help implement the Institute's recently-mandated extension of coverage to the children of covered workers and its assumption of responsibility for primary health care coverage for the members of cooperatives. IPSS will also require technical assistance to increase its collection of revenue within current contribution rates, and to improve its financial management so that it can reach fiscal stability and control costs.

Some foreign aid should be directed to the private health sector, to assist in expanding health care coverage under various risk-sharing mechanisms. However, in many of Peru's low-income urban neighborhoods, smaller towns, and rural areas, PVOs represent the major alternative to MOH-provided primary health care. The loose and poorly-defined relationship between the MOH and PVOs needs to be clarified, and among themselves PVOs need to establish more unified standards of care, costs, and user fee charges. By their very nature, PVOs will always be dependent upon charitable support, so international donor agencies should—as a condition of the short-term financial support and technical assistance they provide—insist on long-term commitments from and coordination among PVO parent organizations.

In general, the major international donor agencies recognize the need to coordinate their activities, but in the case of Peru no effective coordination seems to exist—even though the limited ability of the MOH to manage international support funds efficiently makes such coordination particularly important in Peru. Informal consultation among donor agencies will not suffice to bring about a more efficient and effective use of their contributions by the MOH; donors must reach formal agreement on a unified set of objectives, one of which should be to help Peruvian authorities in managing the counterpart funding and financial accounting requirements of their international benefactors. Donor coordination will be even more important if IPSS and the PVOs are also to be targeted for foreign aid.

One potentially fruitful cooperative effort among international donors would be to decide upon geographical or sectorial distribution of their support to Peru along clearer lines than have been drawn in the past. If Peruvian authorities were obliged to deal with only one major donor for each geographical area—or one for each major health sector institution (the MOH, IPSS, and PVOs)—the overall efficiency of foreign aid could be improved.

If both domestic and international financing of the Peruvian health sector were to increase sharply during a period of favorable economic conditions, it is quite likely that this "boom" in expenditures would lead to a "bust" in support capabilities during an economic recession. International donors should therefore bear in mind the relationships between their financial support of the health sector and the Peruvian economy's overall performance, the Government's ability to finance the MOH, and the financial health of IPSS and the PVOs. Donors might consider building a counter-cyclical feature into their support agreements with Peruvian health sector authorities: if GDP growth is slow or negative, foreign aid disbursements would be stepped up, while during a period of improved GDP growth, disbursements would be curtailed and made more strongly conditional upon Peruvian Government funding of the MOH and increased collections by IPSS of employer contributions.

International donors have long been stressing the important point that recipients must be capable of covering all future recurrent cost obligations resulting from aid-supported projects. In Peru, however, donors have not been sufficiently insistent that the MOH, in particular, budget carefully for increased recurrent cost obligations. Donors should consider making their aid conditional upon specific MOH commitments to allocate specified proportions of ordinary domestic revenues to facilities maintenance, essential medicines, and other important recurrent costs other than wages, benefits, and pensions.

Finally, at least one of Peru's major international benefactors should provide support for strengthening the country's capacity to undertake major research projects of direct relevance to health sector planning and program design. Work at one or more of Peru's several existing research centers could be assisted with short-term advanced training, technical assistance, and direct financial support for equipment and research-related activities such as workshops and publications. The current political situation in Peru does not make this a propitious time for a major policy dialogue between Peruvian health sector authorities and international donors, but sponsorship of participatory research within Peru—such as that conducted by the HSA-Peru—has proved to be an important contribution to the Government's internal policy dialogue.

APPENDIX A

HSA-Peru Participants

HSA–Peru Coordinating Committee

Luis Carlos Gómez, IRG, Ltd., Senior Health Scientist
Cesar Peñaranda Castañeda, ESAN Representative
David Tejada Pardo, UPCH Representative
Walter Torres Zevallos, PAHO, Project Coordinator
Dieter K. Zschock, Stony Brook, Project Director

State University of New York at Stony Brook (SUNY)

a) Faculty and Staff

Ethel R. Carrillo	Economist
Paul J. Gertler	Economist
Luis Locay	Economist
Gloria Malowitz	Secretary
Edmund T. McTernan	Health Administrator
Warren C. Sanderson	Economist
Lynda Perdomo-Ayala	Administrator
Dieter K. Zschock	Economist

b) Consultants

Judith R. Davidson	Medical Anthropologist
Gary Gereffi	Sociologist
Carmelo Mesa-Lago	Economist

International Resources Group, Ltd. (IRG), Stony Brook

Luis Carlos Gómez	Biostatistician and Sociologist
James Munson	Systems Analyst
Petra Reyes	Health Planner
Maritza Torres	Social Worker
Giuliana Mavila	Librarian

Pan American Health Organization (PAHO)

a) HSA-Peru Project Staff

Marco Antonio Ayres	Economist
Julio Castañeda Costa	Medical Doctor
Teresa Ciudad de Iglesias	Psychologist
Ela Díaz de Venturo	Nurse
Olga Diez	Secretary
Alfredo Filomeno	Sociologist
Nelly Gálvez de Llaque	Pharmacist
Noemí Montes	Economist
Luis Olivera Cárdenas	Anthropologist
Susana Cavassa de Pinedo	Secretary
Héctor Ramos Salazar	Demographer
Walter Torres Zevallos	Medical Doctor
Juan Fernando Vega	Sociologist

b) Advisors and Staff

Eduardo Aquino del Puerto	Medical Doctor
Aurora Estrada Falconí	Secretary
Roberto Badía Montalvo	Medical Doctor
Jorge Castellanos	Medical Doctor
Astrid Debuchi	Architect
Enrique Fefer	Medical Doctor
Guillermo Llanos	Medical Doctor
Philip Musgrove	Economist
Duncan Pedersen	Medical Doctor
Daniel Purcallas	Medical Doctor
Clovis Tigre	Medical Doctor
Carlos Vidal	Medical Doctor

Ministry of Health (MOH), Peru

Miyaray Benavente Ercilla	Nutritionist
Manuel Bernales	Sociologist
Javier Bolívar	Engineer
Edwin Cabrera	Medical Doctor
Lydia Carreón	Pharmacist
Maria Esperanza Castañeda	Architect
Banjamin Cóndor	Administrator
Manuel del Río	Medical Doctor
Maria Estrada Farfán	Architect
Petronio Eyzaguirre	Medical Doctor
Uriel García Márquez	Pharmacist
Ruth Seminario Rivas	Nurse
Cristina Silva Alvarado	Administrator
Eduardo Zapata Salazar	Medical Doctor

Peruvian Social Security Institute (IPSS)

Alberta Arenas Horna	Pharmacist
Marina López	Medical Doctor
Luis Manrique Morales	Sociologist
Germán Martinez Torres-Lara	Architect
Eduardo O'Brien Neyra	Economist
Julia Pineda García	Nurse
Nilo Vallejo Espinosa	Medical Doctor

Cayetano Heredia University of Peru (UPCH)

Luis Benavente Ercilla	Medical Doctor
Miguel Campos Sánchez	Medical Doctor
Diego Gonzalez del Carpio	Medical Doctor
Jorge Silva Leguía	Medical Doctor
David Tejada Pardo	Economist
Mario Zegarra Coello	Medical Doctor

Graduate School of Administration and Management (ESAN), Peru

Nissim Alcabés Avdala	Lawyer
Octavio Chirinos Valdívia	Economist
Susana Madrid Wosan	Engineer
Oscar Millones Destefano	Economist
Dora Luz Paz Castañaga	Engineer
Cesar Peñaranda Castañeda	Economist
José Carlos Vera la Torre	Economist
Rosario Vergara Poppe	Secretary

APPENDIX B

Estimates of Sectorial Coverage and Expenditures

Drawing a composite picture of all health sector expenditures and coverage involves combining the relatively few data in which one can have confidence with estimates that can be defended as being reasonable and consistent. Tables 1.1, 1.2, and 1.3 together provide this composite picture for Peru. In Table 1.1, the expenditure data for the MOH and IPSS are reasonably reliable. In Table 1.3, IPSS coverage refers to the mandated total coverage, as explained in Chapter 9 and shown in Table 9.2. MOH coverage is a reasonable estimate, arrived at by estimating private sector coverage (see below), adding coverage under IPSS and other public sector institutions (parastatals and uniformed forces), and then subtracting the result from the total population. This gives us an estimated total, for the MOH's target population, of 11 million Peruvians who were assumed to be medically indigent in 1984—a figure that coincides with estimates used publicly by MOH officials in 1985. These officials acknowledged that only half of this target population, at most, lives within access to MOH health care facilities.

The rural/urban distribution of MOH coverage is also derivative, arrived at by estimating total IPSS and private sector coverage (which is predominantly urban) and considering the remainder as the MOH urban target population. The definition of "urban" in this context, however, refers to the country's larger urban concentrations, which account for approximately 40 percent of the total population, or close to 8 million Peruvians. The definition of "rural" thus includes the country's smaller towns and villages, where most of the Ministry's primary health care facilities are in fact located. (Officially, the term "urban" includes villages with as few as 2,000 inhabitants—hardly a useful definition, since the socio-economic characteristics of settlements of up to 20,000 inhabitants are predominantly "rural.")

The MOH is thus assumed to cover 2 million urban Peruvians, or about one-fourth of the "major urban" population, yet it is likely that it serves a much larger proportion of this population. This is not a contradiction if one can accept that the coverage estimate refers to the MOH target population of medically indigent, whereas users of MOH health services—particularly hospitals—include many whose coverage (at least for ambulatory or natal care) is presumed to be provided either by IPSS or the private sector. Coverage estimates thus artificially distribute the population among the several health sector components without allowing for the overlapping usage of services.

Private sector coverage and expenditure data shown in Table 1.2 are almost entirely estimates. Note that:

1. Coverage estimates for employer and provider plans and for risk-sharing mechanisms were developed by the coauthors of Chapter 4. Coverage estimates for cooperatives are modified data based on a study by Management Sciences for Health (Bates and Prentice 1983); coverage estimates for PVOs are taken from another MSH study (Keaty and Keaty 1983).

2. Coverage estimates referring to direct expenditures by households for private sector medical services reflect the population remaining after MOH, IPSS, other public sector and all private sector coverage has been added up. This includes 500,000 urban "rich," (see 3.c, below) as well 1,000,000 urban poor and 5,000,000 rural poor residents. The poor must be assumed to be the very poorest in the urban areas plus the majority of rural inhabitants, all of whom are beyond the reach of MOH services and of health care provided by cooperatives and PVOs. While these six million poorest Peruvians use traditional rather than modern health care, anthropological research shows that they *are* allocating some income to paying for such services—often by barter, involving only minimal monetary expenditures (Davidson 1983). It is consistent to include an estimate of payments in the form of barter inasmuch as standard national income accounts also include an estimate of in-kind exchanges and household consumption of self-produced farm output.

3. The private sector expenditure estimates are arrived at by assuming for each population segment in the "coverage" column of Table 1.2 an average annual *per capita* expenditure.

a) For the employer and provider plans and the risk-sharing mechanisms, the *per capita* expenditure is assumed to be US $50, which is about US $20 less than the *per capita* expenditure for medical care by IPSS. For urban cooperatives, the *per capita* expenditure is also assumed to be a relatively high US $20, since cooperatives appear to provide ambulatory care comparable to that provided under employer, provider and risk-sharing arrangements—although they probably provide fewer hospitalization benefits.

b) All urban and rural medical services provided by PVOs are assumed to be US $10 *per capita* for their respective population coverage, equivalent to the *per capita* expenditure for primary health care by the MOH (see Chapter 8).

c) Direct household expenditures by the urban "rich" are assumed to be US $30 *per capita*. This may strike one as low, except for the likelihood that a large proportion of wealthy Peruvians probably obtains major medical services outside the country.

d) Direct household expenditures for medical services by the poor in the private sector are assumed to be about US $5 in urban areas and US $4 in rural areas (including barter). Assuming that the poorest third of Peru's population has an average annual *per capita* income of US $100-200, these Peruvians are spending about 2-4 percent of this income on medical services (including any self-medication with traditional remedies, since they presumably do not have enough monetary income to buy modern pharmaceuticals).

4. Pharmaceutical sales in the private sector have been calculated as totaling US $145 million in 1984 (see Chapter 7). Excluding the six million poorest, an average *per capita* expenditure for pharmaceuticals of US $11 is thus equivalent to about 20 percent of total average health expenditures of US $54 *per capita* for the 13 million who have access to either public or private sector modern health services. Total private sector pharmaceutical sales (see Table 1.2) have been divided between households and health care providers. The US $45 million worth of pharmaceuticals purchased by providers is somewhat less than the total of US $55 million in pharmaceutical products purchased by the public sector in 1984. This makes some sense; private sector providers are estimated in Table 1.2 to have accounted for US $60 million in expenditures for medical services, not including pharmaceuticals. The latter would represent about 40 percent of total expenditures for modern health care in the private sector—the same as what the Peruvian National Statistical Institute (INE) reported based on institutional sampling of private health care expenditures.

5. The data and estimates in Table 1.2 are obviously not intended to be definitive. They are, however, meant to complement and be consistent with the public sector analysis of expenditures in Chapters 7, 8, and 9. Tables 1.2 and 1.3 should be regarded as no more than models whose assumptions can be changed —or, preferably, replaced with real data—to yield different results, particularly for private health care.

References Cited

ANSSA-PERU (Análisis del Sector Salud en el Perú)

1986 (July). Informes Técnicos; Informes Exploratorios. Lima: Pan American Health Organization.

Informes Técnicos:

a. Perfil de Salud de la Población Peruana (Informe Técnico No. 1)

b. Demanda de Servicios de Salud en el Perú (Informe Técnico No. 2)

c. Participación en Salud de la Comunidad en el Perú (Informe Técnico No. 3)

d. Recursos Físicos del Sector Salud del Perú (Informe Técnico No. 4)

Encuesta Simplificada Sobre Planta Física, Instalaciones y Equipos de Hospitales, Centros y Puestos de Salud: Cajamarca y Cuzco (Documento Anexo No. 1)

Inventario de Establecimientos de Salud, Perú 1985 (Documento Anexo No. 2)

e. Recursos Humanos del Sector Salud del Perú (Informe Técnico No. 5)

f. La Problemática de los Medicamentos en el Perú (Informe Técnico No. 6)

g. Financiamiento y Gasto del Ministerio de Salud del Perú (Informe Técnico No. 7)

h. Financiamiento de los Programas de Salud del Instituto Peruano de Seguridad Social (Informe Técnico No. 8)

i. Documentación e Información Sobre Salud en el Perú (Informe Técnico No. 9)

Informes Exploratorios:

j. Diagnóstico del Estado de Salud en la Micro-Región Espinar-Chumbivilcas (Informe Exploratorio No. 1)

k. Estado Nutricional de Niños Menores de Seis Años (Informe Exploratorio No. 2)

l. Utilización de Servicios de Salud en el Perú (Informe Exploratorio No. 3)

m. Condicionantes de la Descentralización Administrativa en el Ministerio de Salud (Informe Exploratorio No. 4)

n. Análisis de Importaciones a Perú de Principios Activos para Medicamentos (Informe Exploratorio No. 5)

o. Consumo de Medicamentos por Niveles de Desagregación en Cuzco y Cajamarca (Informe Exploratorio No. 6)

p. El Sector No Público y la Atención Médica en el Perú (Informe Exploratorio No. 7)

q. Financiamiento del Sector Salud en el Perú (Informe Exploratorio No. 8)

Aramburú, Carlos Eduardo
1983. Tendencias Demográficas Recientes en el Perú: Consequencias Económicas y Sociales. In *Población y Políticas de Desarrollo en el Perú*. Lima: INANDEP.

Barsallo Burga, José
1985 (October). *Ponencia sobre Financiamiento de las Prestaciones de Salud en el IPSS*. Lima: IPSS.

Bates, James
1983. Investigation of the Operation and Utilization of Peruvian Pharmacies. In *Investigation of Health Service Delivery in Three Elements of the Peruvian Private Sector*, Volume 1. Boston, MA: Management Sciences for Health.

Bazán Zender, Carlos
1985 (June). *Logros Alcanzados por el Sector Salud en el Período 1980-1985*. Lima: Ministerio de Salud.

BCR (Banco Central de Reserva del Perú)
1984 (December). *Mapa de Salud del Perú*. Lima: BCR.

Blacker, Augusto
1985 (March). La Crisis Económica. *Debate* 31.

Burns, John O., and Paul Prentice
1983. Overview of Health Services Provided by the Cooperative System. In Management Sciences for Health: *Health Services Delivery in Three Elements of the Peruvian Private Sector*, Vol. II. Boston: Management Sciences for Health.

Bustíos Romaní, Carlos
1985. *Atención Médica y Su Contexto: Perú 1963-1983*. Lima: Escuela de Salud Publica del Perú.

Carbonetto, Daniel
1985. "El Sector Informal Urbano: Estructuras y Tendencias." In Alarco, Germán (ed.): *Desafíos para la Economía Peruana*. Lima: Centro de Investigación de la Universidad del Pacífico.

Carbonetto, Daniel, and Eliana Chávez
1984 (June). El Sector Informal Urbano. *Socialismo y Participación* 26.

CBI (Comisión Bicameral Investigadora del Sistema de Seguridad Social)
1984 (November 16). *Dictamen Final*. Lima: Gobierno del Perú.

CELADE (Centro Latinoamericano de Demografía)
1983 (July). *América Latina Según Tasas de Crecimiento, 1980-1985* (Boletín Demográfico No. 32). Santiago, Chile: CELADE.

CNP (Consejo Nacional de Población)
1984a. *Guía Demográfica y Socioeconómica*. Lima: CNP.

1984b. *Perú: Hechos y Cifras Demográficas*. Lima: CNP.

Córdova Cossio, Mario
1985 (July 9-10). *Seminario sobre Reforma de la Seguridad Social en Perú*. Lima: Universidad del Pacífico.

Davidson, Judith R.
1983. *Private Sector Contributions to Health Care in Peru* (unpubl. report submitted to USAID). Lima: USAID.

de Arregui, Patricia, Flor de María Monzón, and Ida Aguilar
1985 (December). *Problemática de Organización y Gestión en Atención Primaria de Salud*. Lima: Escuela de Administración de Negocios para Graduados (ESAN).

de Kadt, Emanuel
1982. Community Participation for Health: The Case of Latin America. *World Development* 10(7):573-584.

ECLA (Economic Commission for Latin America)
1984. *Statistical Yearbook of Latin America*. Santiago: ECLA.

1985. *El Desarrollo de la Seguridad Social en América* (Estudios e Informes de la Cepal, No. 43). Santiago: ECLA.

El Peruano
1985 (October 28). *Decretos Legislativos Relacionados*. Lima: El Peruano, Diario Oficial.

ENAF (National Survey on Fertility)
1977-78. *Encuesta Nacional de Fertilidad*. Lima: INE.

ENCA (National Survey on Food Consumption)
1972. *Encuesta Nacional de Consumo de Alimentos*. Lima: INE.

ENNSA (Peruvian National Nutrition and Health Survey)
1984. *Encuesta Nacional de Nutrición y Salud* (Unpubl. data tapes). Lima: INE.

ENPA (National Contraception Survey)
1981. *Encuesta Nacional de Prevalencia de Anticoncepción*. Lima: INE.

Galin, Pedro, Julio Carrión, and Oscar Castillo
1985. *Clases Populares y Asalariados en Lima* (ms.). Lima: IEP.

Gálvez de Llaque, Nelly, and Enrique Fefer
1985 (February). *Evaluación Preliminar del Programa de Medicamentos Esenciales de Perú*. Lima: Pan American Health Organization.

Garrido-Lecca, Hernán J.
1984. *Essential Drugs Policy for Peru: An Assessment of the Procurement/Production Alternatives* (Unpubl. ms.). Cambridge, MA: John F. Kennedy School of Government, Harvard University.

Gereffi, Gary
1982. La Internacionalización y la Estructura de la Industria Farmaceutica Mundial. *Economía de América Latina* 9 (2do semestre): 219-228.

1983a. *The Pharmaceutical Industry and Dependency in the Third World*. Princeton, NJ: Princeton University Press.

1983b. La Industria Farmaceútica Mundial y Sus Efectos en América Latina. *Comercio Exterior* 33(10): 879-893.

1983c. Producción y Comercialización de Medicamentos Básicos en América Latina y el Caribe: Algunas Experiencias Nacionales y Subregionales. *Comercio Exterior* 33(11):1008-1017.

1983d. Overview of the Peruvian Pharmaceutical Sector. In Management Sciences for Health: *Investigation of Health Service Delivery in Three Elements of the Peruvian Private Sector*, Volume 1. Boston, MA: Management Sciences for Health.

1985. The Global Pharmaceutical Industry and its Impact in Latin America. In Newfarmer, Richard (ed.): *Profits, Progress and Poverty: Case Studies of International Industries in Latin America*, pp. 259-297. Notre Dame, IN: University of Notre Dame Press.

GHAA (Group Health Association of America, Inc.)
1985. *Managed Prepaid Health Care in Latin America and the Caribbean: A Critical Assessment*. Washington, DC: GHAA.

Grados, Rómulo, Jorge Miranda, and Nelly More
1980 (September). La Pobreza en Lima Metropolitana. *Socialismo y Participación* 11.

Grompone, Romeo
1985. *Talleristas y Vendedores Ambulantes en Lima*. Lima: DESCO.

Guerrero, Luis Alberto
1985 (July 13). David Tejada: Un Ministro Diferente. *Hoy* (Semana Política). Lima: Hoy.

Hall, Thomas L.
1969. Health Manpower in Peru (A Case Study in Planning). Baltimore: Johns Hopkins Press.

HCF/LAC (Health Care Financing in Latin America and the Caribbean)
1987. *Private Health Care Financing Alternatives in Metropolitan Lima, Peru*. Stony Brook, NY: Department of Economics, State University of New York at Stony Brook.

Hogart, J.
1978. Glossary of Health Care Terminology. In *Public Health in Europe*, No. 4, pp. 194-196. Copenhagen: World Health Organization (WHO), Copenhagen Regional Office for Europe.

HSA-Peru (Health Sector Analysis of Peru)
1986a. *Health Sector Analysis of Peru: Summary and Recommendations* (Dieter K. Zschock). Stony Brook, New York: Department of Economics, State University of New York at Stony Brook.

1986b. *Health Status of the Peruvian Population* (Luis Carlos Gomez). Stony Brook, New York: Department of Economics, State University of New York at Stony Brook.

1986c. *The Demand for Health Care in Peru: Lima and the Urban Sierra, 1984* (Paul Gertler, Luis Locay, and Warren Sanderson). Stony Brook, New York: Department of Economics, State University of New York at Stony Brook.

1986d. *Health and Community Participation in Peru* (Judith R. Davidson). Stony Brook, New York: Department of Economics, State University of New York at Stony Brook.

1986e. *Health Care Facilities in Peru* (Ethel R. Carrillo). Stony Brook, New York: Department of Economics, State University of New York at Stony Brook.

1986f. *Medical Doctors in Peru* (Luis Locay). Stony Brook, New York: Department of Economics, State University of New York at Stony Brook.

1986g. *Pharmaceuticals in Peru* (Gary Gereffi). Stony Brook, New York: Department of Economics, State University of New York at Stony Brook.

1986h. *Coverage and Costs of Medical Care Under Social Security in Peru* (Carmelo Mesa-Lago). Stony Brook, New York: Department of Economics, State University of New York at Stony Brook.

1986i. *Health Care Financing in Peru* (Dieter K. Zschock). Stony Brook, New York: Department of Economics, State University of New York at Stony Brook.

ILO (International Labor Office)
1978-80. *El Costo de la Seguridad Social: Undécima Encuesta Internacional*. Geneva: ILO.

1983. *Yearbook of Labor Statistics*. Geneva: ILO.

1984 (October). *Nota Técnica de la OIT: Régimen de Prestaciones de Salud*. Lima and Geneva: ILO.

IMS (International Marketing Service)
1977-84. *Perú: Mercado Farmaceútico*. Lima: Datandina.

INE (Instituto Nacional de Estadística)
1978. *La Población del Perú en el Período 1970–2000* (Boletín de Análisis Demográfico No. 19). Lima: INE.

1981. 1981 Peruvian Census (Unpublished data tapes). Lima: INE.

1983a (June). *Producto Bruto Interno por Departamentos*. Lima: INE.

1983b (June). *Perú: Compendio Estadístico 1982*. Lima: INE.

1984a (April). *La Población del Perú 1980–2025: Su Crecimiento y Distribución* (Boletín de Análisis Demográfico No. 26). Lima: INE.

1984b. *Producto Bruto Interno por Departamentos, 1977–81*. Lima: INE.

1984c. *Boletín Especial No. 7*. Lima: INE.

1984d. *Compendio Estadístico 1984*. Lima: INE.

1985a. (June). *Proyecciones de Población por Departamentos* (Boletín Especial No. 8). Lima: INE.

1985b. (August). *Informe Estadístico: Segundo Trimestre de 1985*. Lima: INE.

INE-MOH (Instituto Nacional de Estadístca and Ministerio de Salud)
1985. *Encuesta Nacional de Nutrición y Salud (ENNSA): Resultados Preliminares*. Lima: INE and MOH.

INE-CELADE (Instituto Nacional de Estadística and Centro Latino-americano de Demografía)
1983. *Estimaciones y Proyecciones de Población* (Boletín de Análisis Demográfico No. 25). Lima: INE.

INE-MOH (Instituto Nacional de Estadística and Ministerio de Salud)
1985. *Encuesta Nacional de Nutrición y Salud (ENNSA): Resultados Preliminares*. Lima: MOH.

Informe de Gerencia (Journal of the Peruvian Institute of Business Administration)
1985 (February). *Panorama Macro–Económico 1984* (Informe Económico No. 5). Lima: Informe de Gerencia.

INP (Instituto Nacional de Planificación)
1985 (July). *División Política del Perú por Departamentos, Provincias y Distritos*. Lima: INP.

IPSS (Instituto Peruano de Seguridad Social)

n.d. *Aspectos Financieros Actuariales: Sistema Nacional de Pensiones.* Lima: IPSS.

1983. *Evaluación Plan Piloto Seguro Social Campesino.* Lima: IPSS.

1984a (March). *Boletín de la Gerencia de Salud, No.* 2. Lima: IPSS.

1984b (September-December). *Boletín de la Gerencia de Salud, No. 5–6.* Lima: IPSS.

1984c. *Convenio de Cooperación Técnica con OPS/OMS para el Desarrollo, Mejoramiento y Operación de los Servicios del IPSS.* Lima: IPSS.

1984d (November). *Estudio Financiero Actuarial del Régimen de Pensiones D.L.* Lima: IPSS.

1984e. *Informe Financiero Actuarial del Régimen de Prestaciones de Salud.* Lima: IPSS.

1985a (September). *El Instituto Peruano de Seguridad Social, Período 1975–1984.* Lima: IPSS.

1985b (August). *Lineamientos de Política de Seguridad Social* (IPSS Division of Planning and Budget). Lima: IPSS.

1985c (September). *Estudio de la Situación Financiera del IPSS.* Lima: IPSS.

Izquierda Unida

1985. *Plan de Gobierno.* Lima: Ediciones PCP.

Jaure, Sebastian

1984 (February). Sector Informal: El Amortiguador de la Crisis. *Actualidad Económica* 64.

Keaty, Charles, and Geraldine Keaty

1983. A Study of Private Voluntary Health Organizations in Peru. In Management Sciences for Health: *Investigation of Health Services Delivery in Three Elements of the Peruvian Private Sector,* Vol. II. Boston: Management Sciences for Health.

Mesa-Lago, Carmelo

1979. *Social Security in Latin America: Pressure Groups, Stratification and Inequality.* Pittsburgh: University of Pittsburgh Press.

1983. *Financing Health Care in Latin America and the Carribbean.* Washington: World Bank.

MOE (Ministerio de Educación)
1984. *Estadístíca de Educación 1982.* Lima: MOE.

MOH (Peruvian Ministry of Health)
1975. *Información Básica sobre Infraestructura Sanitaria.* Lima: Ministerio de Salud, Oficina Sectorial de Planificación.

1977-81. *Producción de Actividades de Salud: Informes Estadísticos de Egresos Hospitalarios 1977–81.* Lima: Ministerio de Salud.

1982. *Oficina de Infraestructura Física: Normas y Guías Técnicas* (Vol. I). Lima: Ministerio de Salud, Oficina de Infraestructura Física.

1983. *Proyecciones de Población por Regiones de Salud y Utilización de Indicadores del Sector, Período 1980–1985.* Lima: Ministerio de Salud.

1985. (Unpubl.) reports prepared by health regions for ANSSA-Peru. Lima: Ministerio de Salud, Oficina de Infraestructura Física.

Muller, Frederick
1983. Contrasts in Community Participation: Case Studies from Peru. In Morley, David, Jon E. Rohde, and Glen Williams (eds.): *Practicing Health for All.* Oxford: Oxford University Press.

OGIE (Oficina General de Informática y Estadística, Ministerio de Salud)
1970-84. *Boletines Anuales de Enfermedades Transmisibles 1970–1984.* Lima: OGIE.

1975-81. *Informes Estadísticos de Defunciones, 1975-81.* Lima: Ministerio de Salud.

1977-81. *Producción de Actividades de Salud: Informes Estadísticos de Egresos Hospitalarios, 1977–81.* Lima: Ministerio de Salud.

Olivera Cárdenas, Luis
1986. *The Presence of Basic Organizations Working in Health Matters.* Lima: ANNSA-Peru.

OPS (Organización Panamericana de la Salud)
1979. *Condiciones de Salud del Niños en las Americas.* Washington, DC: PAHO.

PAHO (Pan American Health Organization)

1975 (September 23). *Programa de Medicamentos Básicos en Perú (CD23/29)*. Washington: PAHO.

1984. *Policies for the Production and Marketing of Essential Drugs* (Scientific Publication No. 462). Washington: PAHO.

1985. *The Economic Crisis and Its Impact on Health and Health Care in Latin America and the Carribbean* (ms). Washington, DC: PAHO.

1986. *Health Conditions in the Americas, 1981–1984*, Vols. I and II. Washington, DC: PAHO.

Pennano, Guido

1981. Economía y Realidad Urbana. *Debate* 11.

Price Waterhouse

1984 (December). *Estudio sobre la Evolución Financiera y de los Resultados de la Industria Farmaceútica en el Perú, Años 1976 a 1983*. Lima: ALAFARPE (Asociación de Laboratorios Farmaceúticos del Perú).

Ramos, H.

1981 (March). *Mortalidad Infantil y Atención Materno–infantil en el Perú*. Santiago, Chile: CELADE.

Salazar, Jorge

De Brujos y Otras Yerbas. *Caretas* 847.

Salcedo, Jose María

1984. El Perú Informal. *Qué Hacer* 31:84.

Sara-Lafosse, Violeta

1984. *Comedores Populares*. Lima: Grupo de Trabajo Servicios Urbanos y Mujeres de Bajos Ingresos.

Smith, Michael

1980. Perú: Callejón sin Salida? Reflexiones sobre una Década. *Debate* 6:32.

Stein, Steve

1985. *Health and Poverty within the Socio–political Context of Peru, 1985* (Unpubl. ms.). Dept. of Economics, State University of New York at Stony Brook: HSA-Peru.

Stein, Steve, and Carlos Monge

1987. *Perú en Crisis: Polarización y Respuestas Populares*. Lima: IEP.

Vargas Llosa, Mario
1987. In Defense of the Black Market. *The New York Times Magazine*, Feb. 22, 1987, p. 28.

Vega-Centeno, Máximo, and Maria Antonia Remenyi
1980. La Industria Farmaceútica en el Perú: Características y Limitaciones. *Socialismo y Participación* 10:33-61.

Verdea, Francisco
1983. *El Empleo en el Perú: Un Nuevo Enfoque*. Lima: IEP.

Vieira, Cesar
1984 (November). Alimentación y Salarios. *Actualidad Económica* 71.

Vílchez, Edmundo Cruz
1983 (September). El Movimiento Sindical Frente a la Inflación. *Socialismo y Participación* 23:87.

Westinghouse Health Systems
1985. *Asistencia Técnica en Servicios de Salud*. Lima: Westinghouse Health Systems.

World Bank
1986. *World Development Report 1986*. New York: Oxford University Press.

Zschock, Dieter K.
1986. Medical Care Under Social Insurance in Latin America. *Latin American Research Review* XXI(1): 99-122.

Contributors

Ethel R. Carrillo is associate professor of economics at the University of Lima, Peru. Currently on a leave of absence, she is employed by International Resources Group, Ltd., of Stony Brook, N.Y., under a subcontract with the State University of New York at Stony Brook, as a study coordinator for the Health Care Financing in Latin America and the Caribbean project. She previously worked directly for the university on the HSA-Peru project, and had responsibility for the analysis of health care facilities.

Julio Castañeda Costa is a medical doctor and former senior official of the Peruvian Ministry of Health. He was national coordinator of the HSA-Peru project during its first six months, and subsequently served as a technical advisor to the project. Dr. Castañeda has also worked as a private health clinic administrator in Lima, an experience that served him well in his later collaboration with José Carlos Vera on the field research for the chapter they co-authored for this book.

Judith R. Davidson, a medical anthropologist, is currently a consultant for a health maintenance organization in California. She has extensive field research experience in community health practices and health care financing in Latin America. Following her participation in a study of health promoters in Peru as a consultant to the U.S. Agency for International Development, she took part in the analysis of community participation in health for the HSA-Peru project as a consultant to the State University of New York at Stony Brook.

Gary Gereffi, associate professor of sociology at Duke University, is internationally recognized as an expert on the role of the pharmaceutical industry in economic development. He has consulted for the Pan American Health Organization on the promotion of essential drugs, and participated in the analysis of the Peruvian pharmaceutical industry for the HSA-Peru project as a consultant to the State University of New York at Stony Brook.

Luis Carlos Gómez, professor of quantitative methods and health information systems at the Javeriana University in Bogota, Colombia, directed the National Health Study of Colombia as the last assignment of his 20-year career with the Colombian Ministry of Health. As a part of that work, he designed and implemented the country's National Health Information System. In his role as Senior Health Scientist for the International Resources Group, Ltd. of Stony

Brook, N.Y., Professor Gomez was responsible for the health status analysis carried out for the HSA-Peru project.

Gretchen Gwynne, an anthropologist, is Research Associate to the Health Care Financing in Latin America and the Caribbean project at the State University of New York at Stony Brook. An author and editor of anthropological studies, Dr. Gwynne assumed a major role in editing the HSA-Peru research reports that form the basis of this book. She is currently coauthoring a basic text in cultural anthropology.

Luis Locay is assistant professor of economics at the State University of New York at Stony Brook. With prior research experience in economic anthropology, he participated in a study of household demand for health care for the HSA-Peru project, and was primarily responsible for the design of the HSA-Peru research on medical personnel.

Carmelo Mesa-Lago, Distinguished Service Professor in Economics and Latin American Studies at the University of Pittsburgh, is internationally known as an expert on the role of social security systems in economic development. Prior to his research on the medical care program of the Peruvian Social Security Institute for the HSA-Peru project, Dr. Mesa-Lago had completed a comprehensive regional study of social security development for the U.N. Economic Commission for Latin America.

Steve Stein is associate professor of Latin American History at the University of Miami. Widely known for his work on labor and social history in Peru, he reviewed contemporary social change in Peru in preparation for collaborating with Judith R. Davidson in the analysis of community participation in health for this book. Dr. Stein's research on social change will shortly be published as a book, jointly authored with Carlos Monge, a Peruvian social historian.

José Carlos Vera la Torre, a Peruvian economist, worked for his government's Ministry of Planning and Development prior to joining the HSA-Peru project to analyze health care financing. He was responsible for analyzing Ministry of Health expenditures, and was instrumental in exploring private health sector financing alternatives, together with Dr. Castañeda Costa, under the Health Care Financing in Latin America and the Caribbean project administered by the State University of New York at Stony Brook.

Dieter K. Zschock, associate professor of economics at the State University of New York at Stony Brook, is internationally known as an expert on health care financing in developing countries. As director of the HSA-Peru project, he participated directly in the research on health care financing in the public and private sectors. He now directs the Health Care Financing in Latin America and the Caribbean project under a contract with the U.S. Agency for International Development.

Index